TRADITIONAL CHINESE HEALTH SECRETS

TRADITIONAL CHINESE HEALTH SECRETS

The Essential Guide to Harmonious Living

XU XIANGCAI

YMAA Publication Center
Wolfeboro, NH USA

YMAA Publication Center
Main Office:
    PO Box 480
    Wolfeboro, New Hampshire 03894
    800-669-8892 • info@ymaa.com • www.ymaa.com

20200318

Copyright ©2001 by Xu Xiangcai

ISBN:1-886969-89-2

Edited by Sharon Rose
Cover design by Richard Rossiter

Publisher's Cataloging in Publication
(Prepared by Quality Books Inc.)

Xu, Xiangcai.
    Traditional Chinese health secrets : the essential
guide to harmonious living / Xu Xiangcai. — 2nd ed.
    p. cm.
    Includes index.
    LCCN: 00-109678
    ISBN: 1-886969-89-2

    1. Medicine, Chinese. 2. Qi gong. 3. Alternative
medicine. I. Title.

R602.X89 2001   610'.951
                                 QBI01-200147

Disclaimer:
The authors and publisher of this material are NOT RESPONSIBLE in any
manner whatsoever for any injury which may occur through reading or following
the instructions in this manual.
The activities, physical or otherwise, described in this material may be too
strenuous or dangerous for some people, and the reader(s) should consult a
physician before engaging in them.

Printed in USA.

Editor's Note

Traditional Chinese Health Secrets provides valuable information for beginners, advanced amateurs, and medical professionals. This textbook gives beginning practitioners a comprehensive overview of all of the subject matter and intricacies of Traditional Chinese Medicine (TCM); it offers advanced students practical references, and it provides medical professionals insight into various preventative and curative treatments often prescribed by TCM practitioners.

Traditional Chinese Health Secrets is in no way meant to be a practical, hands-on guide to prescriptive medicine by non-TCM practitioners. All readers seeking such guidance are directed to seek professional education, including TCM diagnostic techniques not covered within this text. As with any medicine—preventative or curative, herbal or chemical, ingested or performed—readers should NOT self-medicate or administer these treatments to others without appropriate education from licensed professionals.

Table of Contents

Chapter 3 Healthcare Independent of Medicines

The Effects of Acupuncture and Moxibustion in Healthcare • Mechanisms
of Acupuncture and Moxibustion • Commonly Selected Acupoints in
Healthcare • Acupuncture and Moxibustion for Healthcare
Ways of Exercising • Types of Qigong Exercises • Principles in Doing
Qigong Exercises
Active and Passive Massage • Self-Massage for Healthcare • Indications
and Contraindications

Foreword

I am delighted to learn that *Traditional Chinese Health Secrets* will soon come into the world. TCM has experienced many vicissitudes of times but has remained evergreen. It has made great contributions not only to the power and prosperity of our Chinese nation but to the enrichment and improvement of world medicine. Unfortunately, differences in nations, states and languages have slowed down its spreading and flowing outside China. Presently, however, an upsurge in learning, researching and applying Traditional Chinese Medicine (TCM) is unfolding. In order to bring the practice of TCM to all areas of the globe, Mr. Xu Xiangcai called intellectuals of noble aspirations and high intelligence together from Shandong and many other provinces in China to compile and translate this text. I believe that the day when the world's medicine is fully developed will be the day when TCM has spread throughout the world.

I am pleased to give it my recommendation.

Prof. Dr. Hu Ximing

Deputy Minister of the Ministry of Public Health of the People's Republic of China, Director General of the State Administrative Bureau of Traditional Chinese, Medicine and Pharmacology, President of the World Federation of Acupuncture Moxibustion Societies, Member of China Association of Science & Technology, Deputy President of All-China Association of Traditional Chinese Medicine, President of China Acupuncture & Moxibustion Society

Foreword

The Chinese nation has been through a long, arduous course of struggling against diseases. Through this struggle, it has developed its own traditional medicine-Traditional Chinese Medicine and Pharmacology (TCMP), TCMP has a unique, comprehensive—both theories and clinical practice—scientific system including both theories and clinical practice.

Though its beginnings were several thousand years ago, the practice of TCM has been well preserved and continuously developed. TCM has special advantages, which include remarkable curative effects and few side effects. It is an effective means by which people can prevent and treat diseases and keep themselves strong and healthy. All achievements attained by any nation in the development of medicine are the public wealth of all mankind. They should not be confined within a single country. What is more, the need to set them free to flow throughout the world as quickly and precisely as possible is greater than that of any other kind of science. During my more than thirty years of being engaged in the practice of Traditional Chinese Medicine (TCM), I have been looking forward to the day when TCMP will have spread all over the world and made its contributions to the elimination of diseases of all mankind. However, it is to be deeply regretted that the pace of TCMP in extending outside China has been unsatisfactory due to the major difficulties involved in expressing its concepts in foreign languages.

Mr. Xu Xiangcai, a teacher of Shandong College of TCM, has sponsored and taken charge of the work of compilation and translation of such knowledge into English. This work is a great project, a large-scale scientific research, a courageous effort and a novel creation. I am deeply grateful to Mr. Xu Xiangcai and his compilers and translators, who have been working day and night for such a long time on this project. As a leader in the circles of TCM, I am duty-bound to do my best to support them.

I believe this text will be certain to find its position both in the history of Chinese medicine and in the history of world science and technology.

Mr. Zhang Qiwen
Member of the Standing Committee of All-China
Association of TCM, Deputy Head of the Health
Department of Shandong Province

Preface

Traditional Chinese Health Secrets is based on the fundamental theories of traditional Chinese medicine(TCM) with emphasis on the clinical practice of TCM. It is a semi-advanced English-Chinese academic work, which is quite comprehensive, systematic, concise, practical and easy to read. This text is designed to give the reader an introduction to the practices and theories of TCM. It is also comprehensive enough to serve as a reference for the TCM practitioner.

Because this text is unique to the Chinese nation, translating it into English has been crucial to sharing the knowledge of TCM practice with the rest of the world.

More than 200 people have taken part in the activities of compiling, translating and revising this text. These individuals come from twenty-eight institutions in all parts of China. Among these institutions are fifteen colleges of TCM: Shandong, Beijing, Shanghai, Tianjin, Nanjing, Zhejiang, Anhui, Henan, Hubei, Guangxi, Guiyang, Gansu, Chengdu, Shanxi and Changchun, and scientific research centers of TCM such as China Academy of and Shandong Scientific Research Institute of TCM.

The Education Commission of Shandong province has included the compilation and translation of this text in its scientific research projects and allocated funds accordingly. The Health Department of Shandong Province has also given financial aid together with a number of pharmaceutical factories of TCM. The subsidization from Jinan Pharmaceutical Factory of TCM provided the impetus for the work of compilation and translation to get under way.

The success of compiling and translating this series is not only the fruit of the collective labor of all the compilers, translators and revisers but also the result of the support of the responsible leaders of the relevant leading institutions. As this text is going to be published, I express my heartfelt thanks to all the compilers, translators, and revisers for their sincere cooperation, and to the specialists, professors, leaders at all levels and pharmaceutical factories of TCM for their warm support.

It is my most profound wish that the publication of this text will help to expand the idea of TCM practice to those individuals interested in this practice.

Xu Xiangcai
Shandong College of TCM

CHAPTER 1

Principles of
Healthcare in TCM

The principles and techniques of healthcare that exist today in Traditional Chinese Medicine (TCM) were gradually developed through thousands of years of study and practice. According to a classic and ancient TCM text, the *Nei Jing,* the ways of TCM healthcare are generalized by the following principles.

> *The techniques and methods are based on the theory of yin and yang and should conform to the natural law. One should keep an orderly life with a proper and controlled diet. One should avoid overwork. Pathogenic wind and other ill factors should be prevented at all times. Essential qi results from serenity and empty-mindedness and will keep you free of disease if you have a sound mind.*

The way of TCM healthcare has been practiced for thousands of years by those who wished to keep themselves in good health. It is under the guidance of these principles that the content and methods of TCM gradually developed and perfected, and they are still highly advocated by healthcare experts today.

1.1 Mental Healthcare

TCM pays great attention to the close relationship between mental activities and health. A TCM theory states that the body becomes an "organic unit" when the body and spirit are integrated. If you wish to strengthen the spirit, you must strengthen the body, and to strengthen the body, you must strengthen the spirit. TCM also theorizes that essence (*jing*), vital energy (*qi*), and spirit (*shen*) are three treasures of one's life. If you cultivate these three treasures, you will live a long healthy life. It is believed that one can be healthy and free from illnesses only when he or she cultivates essence, uses *qi* sparingly, and takes good care of his spirit. This will ensure that he or she will be balanced and full of vigor, with every organ performing its proper function. If the spirit is in a state of imbalance, then the body's essential *qi* will be lost, resulting in various illnesses or even early death. There are many common Chinese sayings that address this situation such as,

> *Those who keep a sound mind will survive and those who do not will die, and those who gain a sound mind will live and those who do not will perish.*

Therefore, according to TCM theory, for the sake of preventing diseases and promoting longevity, it is imperative to keep a sound mind.

TCM theory states that man has seven emotions: joy, anger, melancholy, anxiety, grief, fear, and terror. It is believed that when these emotions are experienced in excess, the *Qi* and blood will be disturbed resulting in pathological changes and bringing about great harm to the human body. As is stated in the *Nei Jing*,

> *It is known that all diseases arise from the upset of qi: Anger pushes the qi up, joy makes the qi slacken, grief disperses the qi, fear brings the qi down, terror confuses the qi, and anxiety causes the qi to stagnate. Anger harms the liver, joy the heart, anxiety the spleen, grief the lungs, and fear the kidneys.*

In short, the loss of balance in the mind and the *qi* will greatly affect your health.

To the TCM practitioner mental healthcare has always been highly valued and applied as a major means of maintaining health and achieving longevity. Mental healthcare serves as a means of building up the body by strengthening resistance against disease.

1.1.1 BEING OPEN-MINDED AND OPTIMISTIC

A Chinese proverb says, "Optimism will help you forget sorrow." It is believed that an optimistic, stable mood and good mental balance calms the body's vital energy and spirit, which aids the circulation of blood and *qi*, thus, improving health. Throughout China's long history, ancient medical texts provide advice on the subject of mental health. For example:

- The ancient book, *Guan Zi,* states, "The quality of one's life depends on maintaining a positive happy state of mind. Anxiety and anger lead to confusion of mind. There can be no mental balance when anxiety, grief, joy, and anger exist. Thus desire should be subdued, and disorder should be checked. Happiness and luck will arrive on their own if there is no such disturbance of mind."

- The *Nei Jing* also points out that "one should strive for tranquility and happiness, while remaining free from anger, resentment, and troubled thoughts. This text also indicates that by avoiding angry moods and a troubled state of mind and by cultivating tranquility, optimism, and happiness, one will obtain longevity with a sound body that is not easily degenerated and a sound mind that is not easily distracted."

- The book, *Huai Nan Zi*, advocates "happiness and cheerfulness," which is said to be a part of human nature.
- The book, *Zun Sheng Ba Jian*, also maintains that "to tranquilize the mind one should have a happy mood."

These texts indicate to the reader that good health is based on happy and tranquil moods. Keeping a happy mood requires that one must have a noble spirit, high ideals, an expanded outlook, a sanguine and lively disposition, and an open and broad mind. As is said in the book, *Ji Zhong San Ji*, "Cultivate a good temperament for the sake of the mind. Tranquilize the mind for the sake of life; avoid emotional extremes and adopt a care-free attitude." Though it may seem difficult, if one can achieve such equanimity, he or she will be safe from unnecessary worries and enjoy an undisturbed mind and a sound body.

Your state of mind also reflects in your ability to deal with problems. Keeping a happy state of mind allows you to tackle problems in a composed manner. The book, *Shou Shi Qing Bian*, says,

> Do not worry about a problem before it actually happens, and do not worry after it happens. Do not cling to what has already passed; rather, try to remain detached and to keep your emotions in check. That is the way to health and longevity.

Within contentment lies happiness, which is important for physical and mental health. The *Dao De Jing* says, "There is no sin greater than discontent, and no error greater than covetousness." Therefore, constant satisfaction knows what contentment means. Additionally, the book, *Zun Sheng Ba Jian*, maintains, "Contentment will bring neither abuse nor danger." Both of these statements express the idea that lasting happiness can be achieved only through contentment. If you think about it, most anxieties and worries result from pursuing and coveting fame, higher status, and material comfort. In the face of such temptations, it is important to stay grounded and realize that there are many people that have less than you do. Such realizations can make it easier for you to refrain from excessive desire and competition. You can than remain content and open-minded, maintaining an optimistic and stable state.

The self-cultivation of one's sense of morality is another important method that helps you to maintain optimism. The self-cultivation of morality is something to which the ancients paid great attention. The cultivation of morality involves devoted attention to things such as moderating desires, remaining content, and being tolerant, kind, and courteous. The ancients believed that a person of great morality was sure to obtain longevity. Through the cultivation of morality a person will cultivate great *qi* which contributes to a balanced mind and a cheerful mood.

Cultivating a variety of interests also contributes to maintaining an optimistic frame of mind. Such interests could include reading, meeting friends, traveling, fishing, playing chess, practicing calligraphy, painting, reciting poetry, singing, playing musical instruments, watering flowers, growing bamboo, etc. According to the book, *Yi Qing Xiao Lu*, "One should always enjoy simple pleasures such as sunshine in winter or shade in summer, beautiful scenes on a bright day, walking cheerfully with a stick, watching fish in a pond, listening to birds singing in the woods, drinking a cup of wine, or playing a stringed musical instrument." What this quotation means is that you should relax your mind, choose and cultivate your own hobbies, and continually increase your interest in life. In doing so, you promote comfortable feelings and a stability of mind, which both contribute to good health and longevity.

In short, open-mindedness and optimism are key factors in regulating the mind. If you can exist in such a way that promotes these factors, then your mind will be balanced and your health will be good.

1.1.2 KEEPING A CLEAR MIND AND REDUCING DESIRE

Through various historical periods, Chinese healthcare experts have always attached great importance to reducing desire and clarifying the mind. They believed this point was important for regulating the mind and prolonging life.

Consider the following excerpts:

- The book *Li Lun Yao Ji* says, "Healthcare lies in reducing desire. Selfishness and desire exist in the mind; therefore, if they become extreme, the spirit and *qi* will be disturbed, and peace and tranquility of the mind will be damaged."

- Lao Zi, the founder of Daoism, emphasized the maintenance of a clear mind and reduction of desire, advocating a simple and plain life without selfishness and desire.

- Ge Hong, a famous physician and world known alchemist from the Jin dynasty, stressed that to adjust one's mind requires purity, modesty, freedom from desire and anxiety, maintenance of essence of life, and simple living with no indulgence in material comforts.

The philosophy of TCM states that humanity has three treasures: essence, vital energy, and spirit. Those that take good care at preserving health will not spend the essences lavishly; rather they will keep hold of spirit, essence, and *qi* by reducing desire, refraining from talkativeness, and avoiding anxiety, respectively. This belief emphasizes that good health can be achieved through reduction of desire and elimination of improper thoughts, thus resulting in the adjustment of *qi* and blood and the preservation of a peaceful mind. Persistence in the practices of maintaining a clear mind and reducing desire will keep all diseases away.

For that purpose, the following three points should be followed:

Controlling the Mind with the Understanding that Selfishness and Excessive Desire Are Harmful to Your Health. The book *Yang Sheng Lun* addresses this issue, stating that one should cultivate an empty and tranquil mind. In doing so, there will be no place for selfishness and excessive desire to take root. He or she should avoid the pursuit of fame and power, because they can harm one's virtue. It is better for the individual to keep out excessive desire, greed, and selfishness rather than suppress them after they have emerged. Once they emerge, they are very difficult to suppress and will harm your ability to create a calm and tranquil mind.

If you can understand the how and why of controlling your mind, then you can help eliminate selfish and improper thoughts. Your mind will naturally become tranquil.

Eliminating six dangers and taking a correct attitude toward personal gains and losses. According to TCM, one of the processes to promoting good health is to eliminate the six dangers: fame, physical indulgence, riches, gluttony, haughtiness, and jealousy. The book *Tai Shang Lao Jun Yang Sheng Jue* tells us to do the following.

- Care little about fame and position
- Refrain from indulgence in entertainment and sexual activities
- Discount riches
- Abstain from greed for food
- Get rid of haughtiness
- Eliminate jealousy

It is believed that if the six dangers are not eliminated, the mind will be filled with anxieties and will not be able to remain tranquil.

Avoiding excessive stimulation of the eyes and ears. Of the five sense organs, the eyes and ears are two important sensory organs that provide the mind a vast amount of stimulation from sources outside the body. Their functions are governed and controlled by the mind. If the eyes and ears are protected from unhealthy stimulation, the mind and the body's vital energy can remain undisturbed. Lao Zi believed that maintaining a tranquil mind could be managed by keeping desired objects out of sight. Similar thoughts can be accounted for in the *Qian Jin Yi Fang*, which states, "What is important in healthcare for the aged is that they should not listen to anything improper, nor talk about anything improper, nor have any improper desire." The key point here is to remove improper thoughts from whatever you see and hear.

In order to control one's personal desire, the ancients came up with some specific measures, such as:

- Cultivating a clean conscience
- Acquiring knowledge of what is to be respected and what is to be distanced
- Developing the ability to be resolute and to detect errors

These measures have positive significance in suppressing desire and calming the mind.

1.1.3 CONTROLLING JOY AND ANGER

Everybody experiences joy and anger, but too much of either is harmful. The book *Ling Shu* says, "Those overjoyed have their minds distracted rather than preserved. Those extremely enraged have their minds confused rather than calmed." Therefore, many of the ancients upheld the measure of preserving a sound mind and vital energy by controlling joy and anger. The *Nei Jing* lists controlling joy and anger as one of the most important measures in healthcare. The book *Peng Zu She Sheng Yang Xing Lun* states "Excessive joy or anger makes it impossible for the spirit to be in its proper position." This excerpt means that too much joy or anger will disturb the mind and cause the vital energy to be scattered, dispersed, and upset rather than being preserved and calm. Uncontrolled joy and anger may also injure one's viscera and the balance of *yin* and *yang* thus causing various diseases.

Suppressing Joy. Joy itself brings about a cheerful mood; however, excessive joy can bring harm to your health. The ancients believed that excessive joy weakens *qi* and injures the heart. Joy in excess can cause you to become over-excited. If a body remains in an over-excited state for a period of time, hypertension and heart disease can occur and become life threatening.

You should learn to regard the events in your life calmly and to judge any matter in an objective and rational way. In this way, strong and transitory emotions can be avoided, which promotes long-lasting happiness and a stable and harmonious state of mind.

Controlling Anger. Of the seven emotions, anger is the most harmful. Anger diverts *qi* and injures the liver. Because controlling anger is so important, it has been written about in many important ancient texts. The book, *Hong Lu Dian Xue*, states, "Anger and rage should be avoided. If *qi* is not confluent, the flow in the channels cannot be regulated. If the *qi* is not regulated, harmony will be disturbed. Anger disrupts the confluence of *qi*." The book *She Sheng San Yao* says, "When one flies into a rage, the *Qi* becomes tough, diverted, disordered, and dispersed rather than gentle, fluent, stable and consistent." The book *She Sheng Yao Lu* says, "Intense anger injures the eyes and dims the sight. Too much anger will disturb all the channels, wither the hair, and weaken the tendons. Those who get angry easily tend to exhaust their spirit; their illness is hard to cure, and their *qi* drains away with each passing day; hence, they will not be able to enjoy longevity." These ancient texts indicate that anger is one of the major causes of accelerated aging and geriatric diseases.

Since anger creates such great harm to the body, you must try to refrain from it or keep it in check. In doing so you must first train your temper and cultivate your mind. During your daily activities try to keep your mind calm and controlled. A famous physician from the Tang dynasty, Sun Simiao gives the following advice: "I say little while others talk a lot. I remain tranquil while others get entangled in affairs. I keep my temper while others lose it. I refrain from feeling troubled by staying away from improper affairs, and I do not follow vulgar custom, so as to reach the state of empty-mindedness."

It would be impossible for anyone to completely avoid stimulation of his or her emotions. However, you can control the effects that your emotions have on your body. Sun Simiao held, "No one can be free from troubled thoughts, but they should be dispelled. When one gets angry, he should make timely effort to comfort himself and dispel his worried thoughts so as to minimize their ill effects on health."

The ancients advocated tolerance and forbearance and regarded them as a person's virtues, which are, in effect, important measures for checking anger.

1.1.4 ABSTAINING FROM TOO MUCH WORRY

Worry is one of the activities of the spirit. Everybody has something to worry about. However, excessive worry will cause anxiety, which will hurt your spirit and can shorten your life. The book *Ling Shu* also says, "Too much anxiety injures the spirit." While the book *Peng Zu She Sheng Yang Xing Lun* says, "Hard and continuous worry will lead to destruction of the spirit." It is believed that the heart houses the spirit; therefore, when the heart is not disturbed, the spirit will be tranquil. When the heart is agitated, the spirit will become exhausted. Since the spirit is the master of the limbs, a sound spirit will bring about a sound body, which in turn will bring about longevity. A sound spirit is brought about by worrying less, desiring less, eliminating disturbing ideas, and resisting all encroachment. The relationship between worry and spirit is similar to the one between fire and oil. The more one worries, the weaker his spirit will become, just as the more the fire burns, the less oil there is to fuel it. Your body expends a lot of energy when you worry excessively. Through continued worry, the body will become extremely exhausted.

We must be open-minded and take a realistic attitude when analyzing and dealing with every day affairs. When it is difficult to free yourself from worry, divert you attention to other things. As time passes, you will worry less.

1.1.5 REFRAINING FROM GRIEF, SORROW, AND MISERY

The great ancient poet, Su Dongpo, from the Song dynasty said, "Man has his grief and happiness just as the moon has its different phases, dark and bright, full and crescent." The ancient people carefully noted the influence that grief, sorrow, and misery have on health. The book *Huai Nan Zi* states, "Too much sorrow and misery lead to illness. Those in grief cannot fall asleep in bed, nor get pleasure even from their best food, nor enjoy music and dance."

Anxiety and grief injure the heart-*qi* and, consequently, the health. It is, however, difficult to avoid anxiety and grief during your lifetime, but you can learn to subdue them.

One should first cultivate the characteristic of open-mindedness so as to refrain from attachment to material gains. This will keep you from grieving over personal loss when it happens. You also need a strong will to overcome sentimentality.

Good friends are important as well. A treasured friendship can replace regret and hatred and heal the old wounds of the mind. Such a friendship can provide sincere help, consolation, and encouragement. These can be magic weapons for eliminating grief and anxiety. When your life is free from anxiety and grief, you will find food tasty, sleep restful, and recreation enjoyable.

1.1.6 AVOIDING TERROR AND FEAR

Terror and fear, no matter what the degree, are abnormal mental activities. Terror means panic, which is mainly caused by outside factors such as sudden stimulation. Terror disperses and disorders the spirit and *qi*. Fear means apprehension, which is mainly caused by inner factors such as dread and uneasiness. Fear depresses the spirit and impairs *qi*. The *Nei Jing* maintains, "Fear depresses *qi*, while terror disorders *qi*." Terror and fear not only harm one's spirit and health and cause disorder of the *qi*; they also hinder normal physiological functions.

It is also believed that through exposure to fear and terror, an embryo can contract disease. Qi Bo, one of the greatest founders of TCM, explained that such disease is called embryopathia. The embryo can contract this disease when the mother experiences a great fright. This causes the *qi* to stay up in confusion and thus plants epilepsy in the infant.

Those who have a weak personality should not travel alone at night or walk alone through thick forests, mountains, or other deserted places. Additionally, attention should be paid to the training of your will so that you can be free from unnecessary panic, which will allow you to maintain mental peace and tranquility.

1.2 Dietetic Healthcare

Food provides nutrients for the maintenance of bodily function and and growth. Good dietary practices insure your health and longevity. Through the years, TCM has developed systematic theories, principles, and methods that have contributed a great deal to the health and longevity of the Chinese people. As early as the Zhou dynasty, "diet doctors" held official positions. Such doctors were responsible for the medical treatment of their patients through proper diet. During the Wei, Jin, and Northern and Southern dynasties, a book entitled *Shi Jing* (*The Classic on Diet*) systematically defined the nourishing functions of food. Sun Simiao, writer of the *Qian Jin Yao Fang*, held the view that the medical treatment function of diet must never be neglected. He stated "Proper food can beat back pathogenic factors, as well as tran- quilize *zang* and *fu*, inspire the mind, and strengthen blood and *Qi*."

The *Yang Sheng Lu* theorizes two methods of healthcare:

1. To keep a sound mind by cultivating one's character

2. To keep fit through proper diet, with the latter as the basis

Later, during the Song dynasty, dietetic healthcare was developed into a branch of science.

Dietetic healthcare plays an important part in longevity. The study of it covers a wide field and is rich with content. Many of the theories and methods developed within this field of study are highly scientific and of great value to all that choose to follow them.

1.2.1 CHOOSING A SIMPLE AND LIGHT DIET

Chinese healthcare experts have always advocated light and simple diets. They believe that such diets can prevent diseases, strengthen the body and prolong life. Consumption of heavy, greasy, and sweet foods over a long period of time produces heat, phlegm, and dampness within the body and tends to cause illness. The *Nei Jing* says, "Heavy and greasy food causes a change that may result in serious illness." In the book, *Yang Sheng Lun*, a comparison was made between the different diets of southern and northern people. In north China, the people are habitually frugal. They consume pickled vegetables and soybean sauce as their main dishes. They suffer less from illness and live longer than those in the south, even though the southern people live areas where all kinds of savory food from both land and sea are available.

Sun Simiao said, "One should cut down on quality food and delicacies and rely mainly on economical food." He also maintained that the diet for the old should mainly consist of non-heavy, lightly salted food such as barley, wheat, and non-glutinous rice. He was a strong advocate of eating less meat and more rice.

Simple and light foods consist of grain and vegetables. Through hundreds of years of research and practice the ancients concluded that such foods aid in resisting disease. Modern research has proven that intake of excess fat in the body may cause the accumulation of fat clinging to blood vessels, thus, promoting arteriosclerosis that will most probably causes hypertension and coronary heart disease. These diseases are often the main cause of death among old people. It is, therefore, quite necessary to control the intake of animal fat and high cholesterol food. Thus TCM maintains that a diet that contains much more of a variety of grains and vegetables than meats has scientific basis.

In addition to a vegetarian based diet, the ancient sages also advocated a diet consisting of food that was mild in taste. They felt that tastes, especially saltiness, should not be too strong. The *Nei Jing* states, "Too much salt will enlarge bones but shrink muscles, exhaust *qi,* and, in particular, depress the heart-*qi.*" The book, *Lao Lao Heng Yan*, adds, "Dishes cannot be prepared without salt, but its amount must be controlled, and the taste of saltiness must be mild so that food may keep its natural flavor and quality. Blood congeals and dries when it meets with salt." Chen Jiru, the author of *Yang Sheng Fu Yu*, explained from his own experience that the intake of too much salt injured the body whereas food with mild taste prolonged life. He felt that people living in the palace lived a short life partly because their food was too salty and the taste too strong. He took examples of three elderly people who, throughout their lives, had rarely taken salt and mainly consumed mild foods; they enjoyed excellent health well into their eighties. Modern researches have discovered that many diseases such as hypertension, arteriosclerosis, heart disease, cirrhosis, apoplexy, and kidney diseases are all connected, to some extent, with excessive intake of salt. The diseases mentioned above are all detrimental to health. Therefore, TCM theory maintains that diets that consist of mild foods and are low in salt help to prolong life.

1.2.2 SEASONING FOOD WITH THE FIVE TASTES PROPERLY

Diets that consist of foods that harmonize the five tastes will result in promotion of the *qi,* blood, and good health. The five tastes are: sour, sweet, bitter, acrid, and salty. If the *qi* and blood are not properly coordinated with the five tastes, the *qi* and blood will be harmed, and one's life span will be shortened. The *Nei Jing* states repeatedly that one must have a fixed diet and that one must arrange the five tastes carefully. It also points out that careful mixture of the five tastes will strengthen the bones, make the tendons flexible, promote the circulation of blood and *qi,* and keep the skin and muscles in good condition.

Eating a Balanced Diet. The ancient Chinese realized that different foods contain different nutrients. They understood that only through a balanced diet could the body get the necessary nutrients to satisfy the needs of its various physiological functions.

TCM theory holds that a balanced diet should consist of grains, fruits, vegetables, and meats. Grains should be the staple food because they contain carbohydrates that supply the human body with necessary heat and energy. Fruits, meat of domestic animals, and vegetables are considered secondary food. Fruits and vegetables provide fiber, minerals and various vitamins, which are also indispensable in the metabolic process. Domestic animals such as pigs, cattle, sheep, and chickens provide the human body with necessary proteins, fat, and amino acids. Protein is a major source of amino acids, the material used to form tissue cells. Fat provides heat while amino acid is even more necessary for metabolism. While this type of diet promotes balance, it also advocates variety so that one does not become dependent upon one particular type of food.

Adjusting the Five Tastes Rationally. As mentioned earlier, the five major food tastes are sour, sweet, bitter, acrid and salty. Each taste promotes a different action and effect on the body. The five tastes should be adjusted in a way that so that balance between them is promoted. One should avoid excess or bias toward any one taste because such imbalance can be detrimental to your health. For example, excessive sour can harm the liver-*qi* and exhaust the spleen-*qi*. Salt in excess enlarges bones, shrinks muscles, and suppresses the heart-*qi*. Excessive sweet disturbs the heart-*qi* and causes an imbalance in the kidney-*qi*. Excessive bitter leads to weakness of the spleen-*qi* and fullness of the stomach-*qi*, and excessive acrid brings about relaxation and debility of tendons and vessels, which, in turn, causes depression of the spirit. Because each of the five tastes links via the internal channels (paths of acupoints) to a particular organ, bias toward a particular taste can harm that particular organ and cause disease. TCM theory believes that after the five tastes have entered the stomach, each then affects its corresponding organ. Sour tastes affect the liver, bitter the heart, sweet the spleen, acrid the lungs and salty the kidneys. As a rule, a long practice of a diet with properly balanced tastes will strengthen the body's *qi*; otherwise, the *qi* will be impaired and trouble will ensue.

In addition to causing harm to the respective organs, excessive tastes will also cause visible pathological changes such as the following:

- Excessive consumption of salt will thicken the blood in the vessels and give rise to change of skin color.
- Excessive consumption of bitter will dry the skin and cause the hair to thin.
- Excessive consumption of acrid will tighten tendons and weaken fingers and toes.
- Excessive consumption of sour will cause a person to grow fatter.
- Excessive consumption of sweet will make the bones ache and the hair fall out.

To maintain a diet that keeps the five tastes in balance, we must:
- Select foods so as to balance the five tastes.
- Regulate the tastes by means of cooking.

This will making full use of the tastes' mutual checking and promoting functions, thus preventing malnourishment and promoting good health.

1.2.3 DINING AT REGULAR TIMES AND CONTROLLING FOOD INTAKE

Dining at regular times and controlling the amount of food that you eat is an important part of TCM healthcare. TCM maintains that you should eat at fixed times on a regular schedule and control the amount of food that you eat. In doing so, there will be no excessive hunger or fullness caused by excessive eating or drinking.

Keeping Regular Dining Hours. The Chinese have long practiced eating three meals a day, with an interval of five hours between each meal. This would seem quite logical since it takes at least four or five hours to digest the food that you eat at each meal. The morning meal is eaten at approximately 7 A.M., the afternoon meal at approximately noon, and the evening meal at approximately 6 P.M. The book, *Lü Shi Chun Qiu*, says, "One is sure to be safe from diseases if he (or she) keeps regular dining hours." This advice was written and followed over two thousand years ago.

Although TCM theory emphasizes eating at regular intervals, it also maintains that an individual eat according to his or her own hunger and thirst. Hunger and thirst may be felt at different times depending on the activity or work schedule of an individual. Thus, although TCM states that you should eat on a schedule, that schedule will vary from person to person. It is important that you be consistent and try to balance your eating schedule with the amount of food that you eat.

It is not only when you eat that is important but how much you eat as well. TCM holds the view that being either too full or too hungry can harm your health. The general rule is eat "neither too much nor too little." The *Nei Jing* says, "Taking no food for half a day will decline the *qi*, and taking no food for a whole day will exhaust the *qi*. Eating twice as much as you require, however, will injure the spleen and the stomach." It is believed that hunger injures the spleen. In contrast however, overeating harms the *qi*. Because the spleen depends on food, hunger will cause insufficiency of the spleen due to a lack of food supply. Furthermore, if you overeat, the spleen will become stuffy, and the *qi* that normally flows through it will stagnate. To avoid this situation (which can be harmful to your health), it is important to eat when you are hungry but not in excess. With this in mind, it is believed that it is advisable to eat more small meals each day—including the three primary meals described above—rather than a few large ones to balance this situation. In doing this, one should maintain a regular schedule and regulate his or her food so that the body remains in a semi-hungry and semi-full state. The *Nei Jing* says, "*Yang qi* is strong at noon but declines at sunset, so it is advisable to have a big breakfast. One should eat less in the afternoon and even less in the evening."

The ancient Chinese healthcare experts believed that controlling food intake is of especially great importance to old people. They also believed that eating less food results in longevity. The principle of lower intake, developed by the ancients, agrees with dietary physiological reality and is of great scientific value. Modern medicine has proved that constant excessive intake of food overburdens the stomach and intestines. It causes an insufficient supply of digestive fluids resulting in indigestion and concentrates too much blood in the stomach and intestines. Thus, major organs like the heart and brain will have a short supply of blood, and this, in turn, causes lassitude and mental exhaustion. Moreover, it may lead to obesity due to the accumulation of fat, which may give rise to diseases such as hypertension, coronary disease, and diabetes. Many scholars maintain that long and constant overloading of the stomach causes an early deterioration of health and can shorten one's life.

1.2.4 REGULATION OF THE TEMPERATURE OF FOOD

Among the other aspects of dietary regulations, the ancient Chinese felt it important to regulate the temperature of food. The book *Zhou Li* indicates that food should be warm like spring weather. Soup should be hot like the weather in summer. Food pickled in soy sauce should be cool like the weather in autumn, and drinks should be cold like the weather in winter. What should be emphasized is that the above-mentioned regulating principle does conform to practical necessity, and it is still being observed even to the present. The ancient Chinese also had a clear understanding about the danger of foods that were extreme in temperature and how such foods affected the organs of the body. The medical classics point out that food that is too hot or too cold can harm the *fu* or *yang* organs. Hot foods can harm the bones while cold food can harm the lungs. The temperature should be regulated so as not to hot to scald the lips or so cold as to hurt the teeth. Food that is excessively hot and cold should not enter the stomach lest it disorder the proper functions of the stomach and spleen.

Modern medicine shows that frequent intake of hot food damages the mucous membrane in the mouth and esophagus, generating corresponding diseases, while excessive intake of cold or raw food can impair the digestive function of the stomach and spleen and, thus, can cause gastrointestinal diseases. Therefore, regulating the temperature of food is of great significance regarding the maintenance of health and should be carefully observed.

1.2.5 FOLLOWING PROPER METHODS OF CLEANLINESS

Clinically, many diseases of the digestive tract such as dysentery and intestinal parasitosis are caused primarily by dirty and unclean food. Although the ancients were not yet aware of such pathogenic organisms, they had already recognized the danger of unclean food to health.

The ancient Chinese guarded closely against unclean food. They maintained that dirty and spoiled food must never be eaten. The book, *Lun Yu*, written by disciples of Confucius during the Warring States Period (476 B.C.–221 B.C.), cautions, "Rotten fish, decaying meat, and food with hideous color or smell must not be eaten." Additionally another ancient text states: "Meat and fish that dogs will not eat and birds will not peck should not be eaten. Meat with red spots should not be eaten. Squashed food kept for many days is harmful to health if eaten. Fruit fallen to ground and bitten by worms or ants should never be eaten."

1.2.6 FOLLOWING SOME INSTRUCTIONS IN DIET

In the practice of dietetics, there are some principles that are advocated and some that are to be avoided. The ancients had principles and advice in many respects concerning diet, such as the proper time, rate, amount, taste, property, and cold-heat factor of food.

The book, *Qian Jin Yi Fang*, notes, "Without the knowledge of correct diet, one cannot enjoy good health." It should go without saying that proper knowledge of what is right or wrong concerning diet has great significance and importance in healthcare. Almost all the discussions on diet in TCM are within the scope of dietetic instructions. Instructions for following these principles can be divided into two parts: instructions in methods of dining and instructions for choosing proper beverage.

Methods of Dining

TCM theory concerning dining methods focuses first on the instructions concerning methods to be adopted at the time of dining and those after dining.

Do's and Don'ts during Eating:
1. **Dining with Concentration of Mind.** It is believed that you should concentrate the mind on the meal when dining rather than become distracted by thinking, talking, or reading because such distractions can affect the taste and hamper the digestion and assimilation of food.
2. **Dining in a Relaxed and Cheerful Mood.** Dining in a good mood helps digestion and assimilation, whereas anxiety, depression, and anger are harmful to your health. It is believed that when you are anxious or angry you should not eat, as the stomach tends to favor tranquility and cheerfulness and the spleen favors music. Thus, music is of great benefit to the digestion and assimilation of food as well. It was also believed that soft and gentle music and a cozy and tidy environment

serves as a benign stimulation that may regulate the digestive function through the central nervous system. Noise, messy environments, and bad smells may affect one's mood and, consequently, one's digestion and health. Thus, for the best possible situation for good health and proper digestion, dine when you are in a relaxed and cheerful mood.

3. **Chewing the Food Thoroughly.** Ancient Chinese medical texts saw the importance of thoroughly chewing food long ago. They urged an individual to chew food thoroughly and swallow it gradually. By doing so both digestion and assimilation were aided.

Dos and Don'ts after a Meal. The ancient Chinese emphasized healthcare after a meal as well as during it. Some statements and discussions concerning this subject are reasonable and practical, having both general significance and considerable scientific value.

1. **Walking Slowly.** It was believed that, following a meal, one should take a walk in order to aid digestion. Walking helped to circulate the qi and the essence of the food through the body. Thus, elderly people in ancient times always took a walk after a meal as a carefree pastime.

   The ancients were opposed to the practice of fast walking and intense movement after a meal. They felt that such movements could injure the organs due to their state of fullness of qi after the meal.

2. **Rubbing the Stomach.** Rubbing the stomach after meal will assist digestion. The book, *Qian Jin Yao Fang,* instructs, "After taking a meal or a snack, one should help digest it by rubbing the stomach with warm hands and by walking outdoors a few dozen paces." It is believed that rubbing the stomach after eating helps the stomach to digest the food, thus aiding in assimilation of the food that was ingested.

   It was also felt that sleeping after a meal could harm you health because lying down would hold the food back in the stomach so that it would not be properly digested.

3. **Choosing Proper Beverages and Drinking in a Proper Way.** The main beverages popular in China are tea and wine. The amount that you drink and the time that you drink is closely observed.

Discussion on Tea Drinking

China is the native land of tea. As early as in the fourth century B.C., tea was already used as a drink in China. In many ancient books, such as the *Shi Jing*, the *Er Ya*, and the *Shen Nong Shi Jing*, descriptions and records about tea can be found. Lu Yu wrote the first book ever written specifically focused on the subject of tea during the Tang dynasty (A.D. 618–905). The benefit of tea to health has long been highly valued. Tea is not only a popular drink among the Chinese, but it is enjoyed by more and more people internationally as one of the three main drinks in the world (the other two being coffee and cocoa). The ancients long ago recognized the role of tea. It was believed that tea could aid one's mind, combat listlessness, invigorate one's body, reduce one's weight, counteract the bad effect of heavy food, and dispel phlegm. With so many advantages, tea drinking is indeed a daily necessity to all.

Modern medical research has proved that tea contains cellulose, colloid, chlorophyll, various alkaloids, vitamins, flavonoids, tannins, ergosterol, volatile oil, hydrochloric acid, thiamine, folacin, protein, and minerals. Drinking tea can refresh the brain, get rid of fatigue, improve memory, prevent cavities, improve eyesight, lower blood-lipids, prevent hypertension, and act as a diuretic.

Although drinking tea has many advantages, it may also bring some detriment to health if drunk excessively or improperly.

Drinking Tea in Appropriate Amounts. It has been found that improper tea-drinking reduces fat in the body and causes cold deficiency in the lower *jiao*. Modern medicine has proven that excessive drinking of strong tea will over-stimulate the body, cause heart palpation and lead to precipitant urination, insomnia, and over-hydration. It will also increase the burden on both the heart and kidneys and cause a vitamin B deficiency.

Refraining from Drinking Tea Right Before or After a Meal. The suitable time for drinking tea is during breaks in the day when one is taking a rest rather than just before or after a meal. Tea contains tannin, which when combined with the proteins in food synthesizes albutannin. This substance may make food hard to digest, cause a contraction of membrane in the digestive canal, affect the appetite, or even lead to constipation.

Refraining from Drinking Tea Before Going to Bed. Since tea contains such elements as caffeine, theocin, and theobromin which have stimulating properties, it should not be taken just before sleep. Otherwise, it may affect sleep and rest through stimulation and frequent urination. Drinking tea is not suitable for people suffering from hypertension, cardiac diseases, habitual constipation, and nervous disorders. Because of improper food interactions, it also should be noted that drinking tea should not be mixed with foods such as leeks.

Guidance in Liquor Drinking

Liquor has a long history in China. The *Nei Jing* contains a chapter devoted to discussions on liquors made from grains. Throughout Chinese history, there have been many contributions to the variety of liquor found in China today.

TCM states that liquor promotes blood circulation through the vessels, increases one's appetite, dispels fatigue, and invigorates one's spirit. It can be used for the prevention of diseases and for achieving longevity as well. The number of the varieties of medicated liquor produced in the past is estimated at several hundred. The book, *Qian Jin Yao Fang*, observes, "Drinking two or three doses of medicated liquor in winter until spring begins is a practice which, if it is observed all one's life, will prevent all diseases. Li Shizhen, a great physician and naturalist during the Ming dynasty, adds, "Liquor is a heavenly drink. Taken in small quantities, it warms up the blood, improves the circulation of *qi*, invigorates the spirit, resists cold, dissolves anxiety, and raises one's interest in life." The property of liquor varies depending on the kind. Generally, spirits (a Chinese white liquor) is thought to resist cold and is used for soaking medicinal material. Rice wine is often used as a guiding drug; yellow rice or millet wine can improve blood circulation and suppress pain. Grape wine can strengthen the heart and aid the spirit. Beer is rich in nutrition and capable of nourishing the stomach and helping digestion. Various medicated liquors are used to prevent or cure many kinds of diseases.

Although the amount of liquor and the way that it is drunk may vary according the particular constitution of the individual, there is a general principle for liquor drinking: drink liquor in small quantities, choose a mild liquor, do not mix different kinds, and do not drink it in an abandoned manner.

It is believed that with regard to drinking, attention should be paid to what is known as the "three propers." The "three propers" include proper quantity, proper time, and proper mood. It has been proved through practice that by following these principles, drinking liquor will be enjoyable and beneficial to health. If one's practice is contrary to these principles, drinking liquor will be detrimental to one's body and mind.

Proper Amount. Liquor of any kind should never be consumed in excess or with abandon. Drinking in such a manner can harm one's health and cause diseases or even death. The book, *Yang Sheng Yao Lu*, advises, "Liquor may benefit the drinker, but it may also ruin one's health. When drunk in proper amount, it will regulate the channels and vessels, drive out pathogenic factors, and resist cold. When drunk to excess over a long period, it will weaken one's constitution and impair one's mind. Thus, one must be careful in drinking and keep it under control."

Alcohol, or ethanol, is the essential element of liquor. In some spirits, the percentage of alcohol is as high as 40–60%. Alcohol can harm your health and in excess it can lead to acute or chronic alcoholism. The state of being drunk occurs when the concentration of alcohol in the blood reaches 0.05–0.20%. Constant ingestion of alcohol may cause chronic gastritis and hence malnutrition; long-term practice of alcoholic drinking also causes cirrhosis of the liver. Thus, disease incidence among the alcoholics is eight times higher than that among non-alcoholics.

Proper Time. It is imperative that one should not drink when hungry. The ancients drank liquor only after eating some food first. Drinking liquor on an empty stomach is most detrimental, since the stomach and intestines will assimilate 60% of it in an hour and 90% in one and a half hours with only 10% excreted out of the body through urination, perspiration, and exhalation. If the amount of alcohol contained in the contents of the stomach is greater than 0.5%, it will become harmful.

It is also believed that you should not drink before going to bed. Going to bed drunk is said to injure the heart and eyes through an overabundance of heat, which results in stagnated dampness giving rise to skin and other external diseases. Additionally, it increases fire and excites sexual desire.

Proper Mood. Liquor must not be drunk when one is in improper moods. Such moods include anxiety, worry, and anger. Some people use alcohol to soothe these moods. There is famous Chinese saying that says, "To suppress anxiety with liquor will only add to the anxiety." Although alcoholic drinking may cause the drinker to have a temporary feeling of comfort, the feeling is just temporary. Eventually it will intensify the particular mood that the person is trying to mask.

Furthermore, one should also abstain from liquor drinking under some special circumstances such as the moment before having sex. In such a moment, if pregnancy should result, the alcohol could cause harm to the fetus, seriously affecting its growth.

Moreover, patients suffering from fever, liver trouble, gallbladder disease, angiocardiopathy, cerebrovascular disease, kidney trouble, and serious enterogastric diseases should also abstain from alcoholic drinking.

1.3 Routine Healthcare

TCM has always attached great importance to an orderly life for maintaining good health and has treated this as an important component of the science of healthcare. It is felt that regularity in one's life and work is essential for preserving health both physically and mentally, as well as for achieving longevity. An orderly life involves many aspects, including regular hours for sleeping and rising, a correct way of sleeping, proper clothing, and personal hygiene.

1.3.1 LEADING A REGULAR LIFE

Ancient healthcare experts believed that whether or not one could enjoy health depended largely on whether or not his or her daily life was rationally arranged. They understood that the channels and vessels were affected if there was no regularity in one's life and no restraint in using one's energy. The medical classics taught them that to achieve health and longevity one should take pains to arrange one's daily life properly, be restrained in one's hobbies, and preserve one's vital energy.

Because the natural climate and environment vary with the seasons, a person's physiological functions also change with the changes of the outside world. With this in mind, keeping regular hours for going to bed and getting up in the morning is very important for keeping balance in your body. The *Nei Jing* states that all living things, their birth, and their death depend on the laws governing the change of seasons and the relationship between *yin* and *yang*. Those who go against the law will incur disasters and those submitting themselves to it will keep diseases away. This book also raises a principle concerning health preservation: one should cultivate *yang* in spring and summer, and cultivate *yin* in autumn and winter. It also gives you a timetable for daily life based on the change of seasons. In the spring, you should be late to bed and early to rise, followed by a leisurely walk. In the summer, you should be late to bed and early rise and not feel drowsy during the day. In autumn, you should be early to bed and early to rise and, in winter, early to bed and late to rise. Moreover, one's daily activities should be adjusted to different times of a day, because *qi* begins to grow in the morning and the *yang-qi* culminates at noon and weakens at sunset. This indicates that the increase and decrease of *yin* and *yang* varies with the different times of the day so one should adapt his or her daily activities. The ancients began their activities at sunrise and stopped to rest at sunset and, thus, demonstrated a kind of timetable showing regular hour for daily activities

1.3.2 THE CORRECT WAY OF SLEEPING

Sleeping is not only a major means of dispelling fatigue and restoring one's energy, but it is also an important process for regulating various physiological functions and stabilizing balance within the nervous system. The ancients paid great attention to the proper way of sleeping. They believed that it is closely connected with health and longevity. An ancient poem says, "Were I to meet with the Huashan Immortal, I would ask him for no divine medicine but his way of sleeping." TCM, by using the theory of *yin* and *yang*, established truth to the thought that sleeping is a necessity for balancing *yin* and *yang* and for continuing the life process.

Pre-sleep Adjustment

During the time before you go to sleep it is important to keep a peaceful mind and a calm mood. Unrestrained joy, anger, grief, and anxiety are all capable of affecting one's mind and disturbing one's sleep. It is necessary to eliminate various thoughts and anxieties before sleep to calm down the mind and spirit. The book, *Yan Shou Yao Yan*, says, "It will be much easier to go to sleep if one washes his (or her) feet in hot water before going to bed. One should drive away all anxiety, thinking only of the pleasant things in life or reading some serene and comforting poems so as to broaden the mind and tranquilize the spirit." It has been proven through practice that washing feet in hot water before going to bed does help calm the mind and enables one to enjoy a better sleep.

Controlling the Intake of Food before Sleep. The Chinese ancients emphasized that "One should refrain from eating one's fill late at night, and he or she should not go to sleep right after doing so." The *Nei Jing* counsels, "When there is discomfort in the stomach, sleep will not be peaceful. If one eats his (or her) fill before sleep, it will add to the burden of one's stomach and intestines, and this in turn will affect sleep and harm one's health." In addition, one should, before going to bed, abstain from taking such things as strong tea, cigarettes, wine, and coffee because they also affect sleep.

Doing a Suitable Amount of Exercise. A suitable amount of exercise before going to bed can help stabilize one's mood as well as relax one's body. It was suggested in an ancient medical text that an individual should walk a thousand steps before going to bed every night. When you walk, you exercise your body and you cease to think, perhaps this gave rise to the idea that moderate movement leads to a peaceful mind. A proper amount of exercise before bed can help you sleep; however, intense exercise before sleep is not advisable.

Inducing a State of Quietness. The ancient healthcare experts developed a number of techniques for inducing a state of quietness for those who have difficulty falling asleep. Of such techniques there were two that were commonly used. One method concentrates one's mind on the crown area, counting silently the breath or concentrating on the *dantian*. This was done so that the mind had a place to concentrate instead of wandering. The second method was to allow the mind to travel to distant places in situation, which can also bring one gradually into the state of drowsiness. The method of counting numbers silently to help fall asleep adopted by some people nowadays is, in effect, the application of the above-mentioned technique.

Principles to be Followed during Sleep

Adopting a Proper Sleeping Posture. The position of your body as you sleep directly influences your quality of sleep. The ancient Chinese advocated sleeping on your right side with your body relaxed and your legs slightly bent. It was believed that sleeping on the right side rather than the left would soothe the spleen and regulate the circulation of *qi*. Sleeping on your stomach is not advisable.

Avoiding Exposure to Wind during Sleeping. Various diseases can result if you are attacked by wind-cold pathogens when you are sleeping soundly. To avoid this, do not sleep in open air or direct drafts. It was believed that sleeping in the open air induces stagnation of food in the stomach and, within a month, will cause any such person to be ill, whether he or she is young or old. When sitting or lying down it is also important that the wind not be blowing at the back of the head.

Sleeping Not Too Near a Fire. The book, *Suo Sui Lu*, discussed this subject stating, "One should not sleep with his (or her) head near a fire or it may injure the brain." If you sleep directly near a heat source, it is most likely that the pathogenic fire may cause diseases. You are also susceptible to catching a cold when getting up at night.

Sleeping with the Head Unwrapped or the Nose Uncovered. As is generally believed, wrapping one's head while sleeping hinders breathing. Air is not circulated properly, and inhalation of impure air can harm one's health.

Making Bedding Warm and Pillow Comfortable. Ancient Chinese medical texts also discussed the condition of the bed as important to proper sleep. It was believed that it is necessary before sleep to make sure that the bed is well arranged, firm, and stable with the bedding warm and comfortable and the pillow soft and springy. In some circumstances it is also preferable to select a suitable kind of medical-herb-padded pillow, which was used to prevent and cure diseases. The pillow height should be at the same height as the shoulder when sleeping on your side.

Healthcare after Waking Up

In addition to paying attention to what one does before and during sleep, great care should also be taken upon waking. In this area there are many approaches. One text, the *Lao Lao Heng Yan*, suggests that one should turn and twist so as to avoid numbness in the lower body or aching in the waist. The book, *Zun Sheng Ba Jian*, suggests techniques such as tapping the teeth, doing breathing exercises, ingesting saliva, and doing massage. Such methods are easy to do and are capable of strengthening the body.

1.3.3 ADJUSTING ONE'S CLOTHING ACCORDING TO CLIMATE

Clothing is an outer expression of one's material and spiritual life as well as a means of preserving warmth and preventing diseases. The ancient Chinese understood long ago the close relationship between health and clothing. They emphasized that clothing should vary with the climate and should be comfortable to wear.

Making One's Clothing Suitable and Comfortable

The ancients advocated that food and clothing are two essentials in healthcare. One's desire for food should be confined to the simple and non-heavy while his clothing should be comfortable to wear. It was believed that it was not the glamour of clothing but rather the fitness of it that matters. The size of clothes should agree with the shape of the wearer, while the thickness or layers of clothing should depend on the season. These statements indicate that the ancients emphasized the value of clothing for its practical use rather than its glamorous appearance. The general principle to be adopted when selecting clothes is to see to it that they are light, soft, big enough, simply designed, and convenient to wear. Moreover, the underwear should preferably be made of cotton material.

Changing Clothes According to Climate

Seasons vary according to climate and so should one's clothing. In spring, clothing should be thick since the weather is still cold. In summer days, clothes should be changed frequently, as the weather is hot and sweating is profuse. In autumn, when weather becomes colder, clothes should be added before diseases arise and medicine is needed. During the three months of winter, the heaven and earth are closing;

add clothes only when it is cold enough. Increase the layers and thickness of clothes gradually and not abruptly.

As was stated by Sun Simiao, "One will benefit a great deal both in health preservation and in preventing diseases if he (or she) follows the law of nature to which he (or she) should adjust his (or her) food, clothing, sleeping, and housing."

1.3.4 PAYING ATTENTION TO HYGIENE

The ancients paid much attention to personal hygiene, believing that only through hygiene will it be possible to achieve prevention of illness and good health. They were concerned with such techniques as mouth-rinsing, tooth-brushing, bathing, face-washing, foot-washing, and tooth-tapping; they have handed down many detailed instructions, many of which are quite scientific and still have practical, guiding significance.

Mouth-Rinsing and Tooth-Brushing

Ancient experts in healthcare were aware long ago that oral hygiene is important for preventing diseases of the mouth. They maintained that you should rinse your mouth after a meal and brush your teeth each night. They knew that food that remained between the teeth caused odor and tooth decay.

Tooth-brushing is one of the inventions of the ancient Chinese. They were using tooth powder to clean the teeth as early as the Song dynasty (A.D. 960–1278). During the Yuan dynasty (A.D. 1206–1333), a noted physician named Hu Sihui recorded in his book, *Yin Shan Zheng Yao*, "Brushing teeth with salt in the morning can prevent odontopathy." Additionally, the book, *Jin Dan Quan Shu* states, "Most people today clean their teeth in the morning, but this has wrongly been inverted. Teeth should be brushed at night, instead, for the remains of food that is between the teeth will be cleared away in time to keep them from decaying. Some wise people have their teeth white, firm, and free from decay until they are old just because they have persisted in brushing teeth each night." The book, *Wei Sheng Bao Jian*, however, advocates tooth brushing both in the morning and at night, a rational practice that is popular even today.

Points for Attention on Bathing

The cleanliness of the body is a necessity for preserving one's health. Bathing, including washing the hair and the body, was practiced in China long ago. Some classical works such as the books, *Chu Ci, Shi Ji,* and *Meng Zi,* all mention the practice of bathing by the ancient Chinese, indicating that they had the tradition of taking care of personal hygiene.

In terms of water temperature it was stated that the water for bathing should not be too hot; its temperature should be agreeable to the body.

They also utilized techniques such as a dry bath and a medical bath. A dry bath was a method of rubbing one's hands on the stomach before sleeping at night. A medical bath included bathing in special decoction made from wolfberries. The medical bath was believed to help prevent disease and aging.

The book, *She Sheng Xiao Xi Lun*, also counsels, "During winter, the *yang-qi* stays inside while the *yin-qi* outside; thus, it is not advisable for old people to bathe too often because they usually suffer from the disorder of heat in the upper body and cold in the lower body." Modern medicine also holds that elderly people need not bathe so often, because their sebaceous glands are shrinking, and frequent baths may cause dryness of skin and itching. For the elderly, dry bathing or rubbing the body with a dry towel is preferable.

Ancient texts such as the *Tai Ding Yang Sheng Zhu Lun* and *Lao Lao Heng Yan* discuss the frequency of bathing. It was stated that taking a bath every ten days is recommended except in summer. Frequent baths, are not taught, only make a person feel seemingly comfortable and regulated, but inwardly his or her essential *qi* is dispersed and dissipated. The books also state that one should not bathe when hungry and that wind must be avoided when bathing.

Hygiene of Hands and Feet

Hands and feet directly contact the outside world most frequently, but are the least protected; thus, they are most vulnerable to contamination of various kinds. Hygiene of hands is closely related to the health of an individual. Apart from regular washing of hands and keeping them clean, the nails should also be cut regularly. Those who wrote the text, *Yang Sheng Shu*, believed that the nails were the ends of tendons, and if not cut regularly, the tendons would not be easy to renew.

It was also recommended that one should wash one's feet in hot water before sleeping. This is done to help stabilize one's mind and promote sleep.

1.4 Balance Between Work and Rest

Throughout history mankind has had to work and struggle against nature in order to survive. In doing so, however, one must work within the limits of his or her tolerance and must rest to relieve tension caused by work. This is known as striking a proper balance between work and rest. TCM insists that this balance must have great beneficial effects on health. Moderate work and rest is advocated rather than excessive hard work and too much rest. Healthcare experts through the ages have maintained that imbalance between work and rest is a great taboo.

Imbalance between work and rest is harmful to health in several ways. Internal injuries caused by overstrain may involve not only the physical and mental types but stress that is due to sexual intercourse. Injuries caused by too much leisure will involve either mind or body or a combination of the two.

1.4.1 AVOIDING OVERWORK

TCM believes that overwork may injure the body, causing tiredness and listlessness in mild cases and result in relevant pathological changes in the severe cases. The *Nei Jing* states, "There are five kinds of over-strain that are responsible for internal injuries: Looking too long harms to the blood; lying too long, the *qi*; sitting too long, the muscles; standing too long, the bones; and walking too long, the tendons." This means that keeping any of the above-named postures for a long period of time can harm the body.

The *Nei Jing* also points out, "Overwork consumes the *qi*, which indicates that excessive physical or mental exertion is chiefly responsible. The shortage of *qi* will cause tiredness, lack of spirit, and weakness." For example, fast walking for a long time may put the body and mind in an intense state and greatly consume the primordial energy. As a result, the vital energy will remain in the interior instead of spreading out. You will feel tired, and it will be difficult to continue walking. If you sit quietly for too long the function of the spleen and stomach may slow down. Because the spleen relates to the movements of muscles, sitting for too long will cause stagnation of the spleen-*qi* and will weaken the muscles. Standing for long periods stretches the waist and bones and strains the residence of the kidneys (the lumbus). Since the kidney is responsible for the bones, standing for too long can injure the lumbus and in turn weaken the bones. Lying for long periods makes it difficult for the lungs to carry out their normal function. The lungs are in charge of the *qi*. Stagnation of the lung-*qi* can slow down the circulation of the general *qi*.

TCM has always considered internal injuries due to fatigue to be an important cause of diseases. Modern medical science also believes that when people are exhausted, their resistance to diseases may be remarkably reduced, resulting in a variety of diseases.

According to TCM theory, there are other ways as well to overwork the body. Such ways include excessive diet, imbalance of metabolism, and lack of spirit. The *Nei Jing* discussed these ways as well. "Sweat comes from the stomach when one eats his (or her) fill; from the heart when one is in great terror; from the kidney when one walks a long distance with heavy load; from the liver when one is frightened or takes a fast walk; and from the spleen when one works with rocking movements." The ancient Chinese were very concerned that anything in excess would overwork the body and cause injury. They believed in keeping a proper balance between work and rest.

The book, *Bao Sheng Yao Lu*, taught that those who practice good healthcare would work without becoming over-fatigued. It professed that flowing water remains fresh, while stagnant water is stale. Thus, those who want to keep healthy must keep the blood circulating like flowing water. Moderate work and proper rest will do this. Thus it is important for a person to find a balance between work and rest that is good for one's own body.

1.4.2 AVOIDING IRRITABILITY

TCM maintains that anything in excess can be harmful to your mind and body. Experiencing extremes of any of the seven emotions is no exception. It is believed that subjecting yourself to extreme emotions will harm the mind and body and reduce longevity. The book, *Ling Shu*, addresses this theory:

> *Apprehensions and anxieties may injure the mind, thus making people weak and emaciated with dried hair and pallid countenance. Continuous worry and anxiety may injure intention, which leads to debility of the limbs. Sorrow injures the soul, thus causing the decline of yin and convulsions. Excessive joy may injure the spirit, leading to the withering of the hair. Excessive anger may injure the will, making it difficult for the spinal column to bend and stretch. Being in terror may injure the primordial energy, leading to debility of the bones.*

This portion of the text clearly indicates that an excess of any of the seven emotions may not only injure the mind but the body as well.

TCM proposes methods to keep the mind healthy which include methods of spirit recuperation, including optimism, lower levels of anxiety and lust, refraining from excess joy and anger, abstention from too much thinking and worrying, and avoidance of terror. All of these methods are useful for preventing the mind from being injured.

1.4.3 REGULATING SEXUAL LIFE

Sexual activity is an important part of human life. Several thousands of years ago, the Chinese people began to study the subject of sexual life. Since then, medical scientists through the ages have put forward many scientific views about the influence of sexual life on physiological function and pathological changes of the body.

Long ago, the ancient Chinese discovered that sexual intercourse in excess is harmful to health. The *Nei Jing* cautions, "Some people regard alcohol as tonic, the abnormal way of life as conventional. They enjoy their sexual life after being drunk, which will exhaust their genuine *qi*. So those who indulge themselves in sexual activity will become senile in their fifties." It was believed that overindulgence in sexual activities resulted in a short life span.

The ancients believed that excess intercourse mainly consumed the primordial energy, which is the base of health. The less primordial energy an individual has the more exhausted they become resulting in disease and even death. So as not to exhaust the primordial energy, sexual activities were restricted.

In order to restrict sexual activities to conserve *qi*, TCM suggests the following propositions.

Marrying at a Mature Age. TCM advocates marrying at a mature age. It is considered harmful to your health to marry too young. It is believed that if one marries too young, the primordial *yang* and vital energy may be injured. This will weaken the *qi* and distract the spirit resulting in impotence and other consumptive diseases.

The suggested ages that one could marry at depended on different physiological development of both sexes. It was suggested that it was reasonable for males to marry at thirty and females at twenty. These ages allowed the female sufficient time to nourish her blood and the male time to control his sexual passion.

Regulating Sexual Life. The ancients also offer suggestions to the frequency of the sexual act. It was believed that individuals in their twenties could have sex once every four days, those in their thirties once every eight days, and those in their forties once every sixteen days. Those individuals that were in their fifties once may have sex once every 20 days, and those in their sixties once a month if they are very strong. It is obvious that the frequency of sexual life varies greatly with age. The general trend is that the older a person is the less sexual activity he or she should have.

Modern medicine teaches that the frequency of sexual activity depends on whether the person is still in high spirits and full of vigor the next day. Today, most people in general believe that once or twice a week is normal and adequate. This frequency can bring about a satisfaction that is not harmful to the health.

Taboos for Sexual Life. In addition to timing and frequency of sexual activities, the ancient Chinese also had certain sexual taboos that they felt could be harmful to the body.

It was believed that sexual intercourse should be avoided just after a bath or a long journey, when you are tipsy or drunk, when you are experiencing extreme emotions, and during the times of menstruation and postpartum.

The book, *Shou Shi Bao Yuan*, points out that sexual intercourse when full or drunk may cause a man to be impotent and a woman to have less blood with each period because the blood *qi* will become injured. Sexual intercourse during a drunken state was also believed to consume the vital energy of the liver and intestines and to cause malignant boils to form.

Sexual intercourse that occurs during times of anger was said to make the essence of life deficient resulting in boils, terror, *yin* and *yang* insufficiencies, spontaneous perspiration, and night sweating.

Sexual intercourse after a long journey will cause infertility and, during menstruation, will would cause cold to invade the body, leading to pale skin and infertility.

Of the sexual taboos, there are three that were regarded as most important.

- Do not have sexual activity when under the influence of alcohol.
- Do not have sexual activity when experiencing extreme emotions
- Do not have sexual activity during unusual weather

1.4.4 AVOIDING EXCESSIVE LEISURE

While TCM maintains that an individual should take care not to overwork themselves, they should also take care not to have a life that is too easy and comfortable. Once again balance is key.

When an individual is tired, it is important to get proper rest; however the rest must not become excessive because it can become harmful.

It was taught that too much leisure and comfort can slow down the circulation of *qi* and blood, hold up the channels, reduce the functions of the organs, fatigue the limbs, and thus lead to general deficiency of the body. The ancients noted three ways to refrain from excessive leisure.

The first way to refrain from excessive leisure is physical exercise. Exercise provides a means for the blood and *qi* to move about the body freely. As the blood and *qi* flows through the body it nourishes it and makes it healthy.

The second way is to avoid sitting or lying for long periods of time. TCM believes that sitting for long periods will harm the muscles, while lying for long periods will harm the vital energy.

The third way is to use the brain frequently. The brain must be used frequently so as to prevent the decline of intelligence. This is imperative for old people. The elderly need sufficient information to stimulate the cerebral cortex frequently so that their brains can be supplied with enough blood. Old people should often read books and newspapers and keep their minds active.

In recent years, scientists have used ultrasonic waves to measure the brain functions of people with varying mental activities. They found that those who keep their brains active have well-nourished nerve cells and dilated vessels, which keeps their brains from declining.

1.5 Healthcare by Sports

Sports in healthcare have been a part of the Chinese culture since ancient times. Hua Tuo, a famous physician during the Han dynasty created the sport *Wu Qin Xi* or Five Animal Boxing, which made a great contribution to the development of ancient sports.

TCM believes that participation in sports can keep the primordial energy running within the body and improve the digestive function of the spleen and stomach. Modern medical research indicates that sports can increase the functions of the heart and blood vessels, improve the function of the respiratory system, exert a good effect on the nervous system, strengthen the muscles and bones, and prevent and control some diseases. Therefore, sports are essential to health and longevity.

Exercises can be divided into two types: active (such as labor and sports) and passive (such as massage). Regular physical exercise can keep you fit and let you live a long time.

1.5.1 PARTICIPATING IN PHYSICAL LABOR

Labor creates the world; it is an essential factor for people to survive. Regular and adequate physical labor is also an important form of exercise. TCM maintains that physical labor can build up the body, adjust the spirit, regulate *qi* and blood, relax the muscles and tendons, and strengthen the bones. Physical labor is especially important for those individuals who do a lot of mental work and for old people. It cannot only train the body and improve health, but it can also mould one's temperament and cultivate one's sentiment. At the same time, physical labor can give your brain time to rest, steady your mood, and give you spiritual pleasure.

1.5.2 BRIEF INTRODUCTION TO COMMON EXERCISES

The ancients paid special attention to physical training and created many sports unique to the Chinese nation, such as *Taijiquan, Wu Qin Xi, Ba Duan Jin*, and many others. Many of these sports are still popular in the world today. The following are examples of a few common exercises that are practical and for the most part easy to learn.

Walking. Walking is the easiest and most frequently used exercise. The ancients strongly believed that people should take a walk in the early morning, after a meal, before sleep, or during free time in order to build up their bodies, regulate *qi* and blood, improve the transport and conversion of food, and invigorate the mind. There is a special discussion on walking in the book, *Lao Lao Heng Yan,* which says, "A walker should walk at a leisurely pace, stopping to rest at intervals." It also points out that walking has the effect of relaxing muscles and tendons, strengthening the limbs, promoting digestion, and tranquilizing the mind. It has been proven that walking is a method of exercise that is both beneficial to health and easy to practice.

Dancing. Dancing is also an effective method for building up one's body. According to the book, *Lü Shi Chun Qiu,* "Dancing can promote blood circulation, thus preventing the stagnation of *qi* and the contraction and spasm of the tendons and muscles." Modern investigations suggest that lively dancing can indeed enhance one's constitution and invigorate one's mind.

Dao Yin. *Dao Yin* is an exercise used in health preservation. It combines physical movement and breathing. This exercise has been handed down from ancient times. Examples of this type of exercise include five-animal-mimic boxing and the twelve ways of *Brahman Dao Yin*. The ancients believed that *Dao Yin* combined meditation and physical activity, and thus promoted the flow of the blood and *qi*, relaxed the muscles and tendons, strengthened bones, and relieved tiredness and restlessness.

Taijiquan. Taijiquan or shadowboxing is derived from Chinese boxing, and was developed during the late Ming dynasty. Shadowboxing is a combination of both dynamic and static exercises, which trains the body internally and externally. Shadow-boxing is named after the diagram of *Tai Ji,* which depicts the relationship between *yin* and *yang*. The practice of *taijiquan* helps to balance the *yin* and *yang* of the body to keep it in a healthy state.

After 1949, the Chinese National Sports Committee published diagrams and captions of simplified shadow-boxing, which is easy to learn and practice.

1.6 Healthcare by Conforming to Nature

TCM maintains that the changes of climate and surroundings are closely related to human health. Guided by the theory of the correspondence between man and the universe, ancient medical scientists believed that human beings and the natural environments are in unity. Consistent changes of climate of the four seasons and environments affect not only the body's physiological function but also, under certain conditions, affect the occurrence and development of pathological processes.

If the six factors (wind, cold, heat, dampness, dryness, and fire) change according to natural laws, they will not harm the human body. If the climate changes abnormally, the six factors will become six exogenous pathogenic factors and cause harm to the body. If people do not adapt to the geographical changes, such as moving from the high land to the wet plain, or from the hot south to the cold north, they will develop diseases due to these changes. In order to gain and maintain health, people must adapt themselves to environmental changes and keep away from pathogenic factors.

1.6.1 LIVING ACCORDING TO THE FOUR SEASONS

It is believed that, to keep healthy, people should act in accordance with the changes of the four seasons. The *Nei Jing* says,

> *The yin and yang in the four seasons are the essentials for all things to exist. The reason that the wise nourish yang in spring and summer and nourish yin in autumn and winter is simply for meeting the basic requirements of yin or yang. Human beings, like all the other living things, lead a certain length of life: they neither die young nor live forever. Going against the regular changes of the seasons means damaging the essentials and primordial qi. The changes of yin and yang of the four seasons are essential for making things appear or disappear, for human beings to come into being or pass away. Going against them means disaster, going with them means no severe disasters. This is the way to keep health. The wise will follow it, but the dull-witted will not.*

The following is how TCM treats the four seasons:

Healthcare in Spring. TCM teaches that spring is the season when everything has a tendency to grow and develop and when all plants are in bud and are flourishing. Human beings should conform to the season in daily life. The *Nei Jing* states, "Spring is the season with active force.

In spring everything is thriving. In this season people should go to bed and get up early. After getting up in the morning, they should have a stroll in the court with their hair disheveled, thus relaxing their bodies and invigorating their mind." The *Nei Jing* further explains that those who do not do this may hurt their livers in spring. A troubled liver will in turn suffer from a pathologic change of cold nature in the coming summer.

In terms of diet, it is taught that one should eat more sweet and less sour food. Since it is warm in spring, food should also be cool in nature as well. It is also suggested that you should not drink too much alcohol or eat too much dough from rice or flour, which is hard to digest and may hurt the spleen and stomach. Therefore in spring you should have food that is soft and easily-digested, that is sweet in taste, that is not dry or sour, and that is pungent in taste and warm in nature.

In terms of clothing, it is suggested that you should not wear cotton-padded clothes that are too thin when it is still chilly. Because the temperature is changeable in spring, you should reduce the amount of what you wear gradually. In general, old people are especially subject to a deficiency of *qi* and a weakness of the bones and the body, and can easily be harmed by wind and cold. Because of this it is very important that they adjust their clothing gradually so as not to become ill.

Healthcare in Summer. Summer is the hottest season in a year. In summer all living things flourish, and because of this *yang-qi* is easily expelled. The *Nei Jing* teaches that in summer one should not go to bed too early at night but should get up early in the morning to enjoy the longer daytime. You should be full of energy and avoid getting angry, thus activating the function of *qi*.

During the summer months you should eat less foods that are bitter and more that are acidic in nature to nourish the lung-*qi*. During the late summer or early autumn months, many diseases are caused by too much greasy or fried food, which has the same effect on the body as alcohol and fruit.

The ancients also offered advice for cooling the body during the hot summer months. It was taught that to cool the body down one should enjoy cool at places such as an empty room, a pavilion by the water, or the shade of a tree. They believed that natural coolness is more comfortable to the body and the mind.

During the hot summer months you should also avoid being attacked by coolness so as to prevent pathogens from entering the body.

Healthcare in Autumn. According to the *Nei Jing*, in autumn, all living things are ripe and stop growing. The sky looks higher and the wind is stronger. People should adapt themselves to the climactic features by going to bed and getting up early so as to calm their mind and make sure that their lung-*qi* is kept pure and descending.

During the autumn months it is dry so eating sesame is recommended to moisten the dryness. Eating a gruel that contains *Radix Rehmanniae* is recommended to nourish *yin* and to add moisture as well. Food should be less pungent and more sour in taste so that excess lung *qi* will not suppress the liver *qi*.

You should also adjust your clothing so that you feel comfortable and do not catch cold.

Healthcare in Winter. During the winter months it is cold and everything is in storage. It is important that you keep warm and store up the *yin* essence inside and allow less *yang* energy to be lost. The *Nei Jing* states, "The winter months are such a season that all things hide, water ices, and the earth cracks. One should be in good spirits and maintain *yang*, go to bed early and get up after sunrise, think as if he [or she] had had what he (or she) wanted, avoid being exposed to cold and keep warm but not sweaty lest the *qi* be affected." It was believed that failure to follow the above advice would cause injury to the kidney-*qi* making it more difficult for the individual to adapt to the spring.

With respect to diet it was advised that food should be less sour and more bitter in order to nourish the heart *qi*.

Clothing, it was advised, should be added gradually as the weather got colder. Although houses were heated by stoves, it was cautioned that an individual should not warm his or her hands and feet directly over the stove because it would affect one's irritability.

In short, the ancient medical practitioners made great contributions to human health. Their statements on the conservation of health in the four seasons still have practical and guiding significance today in the practice of TCM.

1.6.2 ADJUSTING THE ENVIRONMENT

Different conditions of natural environment and climate can have different influences on your health. It was observed that people living at the same place under the same climate yet in different terrain had different life spans. The ancient Chinese concluded that those individuals living in a higher altitude live longer than those living in lower altitudes.

A great deal of research material indicates that longevity is closely related to geographical features. Investigations in the *Duan* and *Bama* of *Guangxi* provinces (the famous longevity area of China) show that all the people who were above one hundred years old lived in the countryside, and most of them lived halfway up the mountains. Another investigation in *Hubei* province also shows that of 125 ninety-year-olds, over 96% lived in the countryside. Certainly, this is not absolute, but the result of all the investigations shows that the supposition of the ancient Chinese was on the right track.

Since environment has a close relationship to human health, people should properly adjust it and make it beneficial to health and longevity. The adjustment mainly lies in the choice and improvement of the living environment.

Choice of Environment

The ancient Chinese attached great importance to the choice of environment. They believed that houses built in the lower, wet, and dirty places will cause various diseases, while those built in higher, clean, and dry places made for long and healthy living.

The book, *Bo Wu Zhi*, points out that a house should not be built in a place near stagnant water or a cemetery. It should also not be built in a lonely a place where wild animals such as foxes often hunt. Rather it should be built in a place before a hill, by a river, with crisp air, sufficient sunshine, clean spring water, and green trees. Such an environment should be free of dense smoke and dirty fog, sandy or black dust, dirty mud and water, and loud noise. Generally speaking, mountain areas are preferable to the plains and the country is better than city.

Adjustment of Environment

The choice of living environment is certainly important, but owing to actual circumstances, the chances of being able to choose ideal conditions are slim, sometimes even impossible, especially in densely populated cities. The choice, therefore, is quite limited. It is, however, possible to adjust your living environment to promote good health.

Improvement of a Room. A room should provide a nice microclimate where people can rest, sleep, and be refreshed. TCM states that a room should protect a person from wind attacks, so it should not let wind through it. It should be clean and warm in the winter and cool in the summer. The bed should have a screen on three sides and should not be too high or large and the sheets should be soft and smooth. The ancients were fastidious about the location and height of the bed, the direction that the room faced, and the position of the windows in it. For example, the book, *Tian Yin Zi Sheng Shu*, says,

> *What is a good room to live in? It is not a hall with a large bed and thick bed clothes. A good room should face south with the bed put in the east of it. It is half bright and half dim with moderate*

yin and yang brightness. Too much light in it is harmful to the human body and too much dimness will hurt a person's spirit. The human spirit belongs to yang while human body to yin. If yin and yang are not balanced, one will be ill. The room I live in has windows on every wall. They are closed when there is wind and opened when the wind stops. The room has curtains in the front of it and screens at the back. I put down the curtains when too bright in order to make the light soft and pull them up when too dim in order to let light in. As a result, both my heart and eyes are eased and I feel comfortable.

Modern research also shows that other factors of a room are important, such as volume, height, and width. A room should not be too small or too low. The volume of a room for one person to live in is at least 15m³. The height should be 2.6–3.5 meters and the width should not be over 2.0–2.5 times the height from the floor to the top of the windows. The temperature should be kept within 17–22°C in winter and 17–25°C in summer. The relative humidity should be within 40–60%. Circumstances permitting, one should improve his or her room according to the requirements mentioned above in order to preserve one's health.

Improvement of Surroundings. It is believed that the surroundings of a room—the yard—are closely related to health; therefore, they should be improved and beautified. The ancient healthcare experts attached great importance to the living surroundings. Most of their houses were situated in places where there were green hills, clean water, and plenty of sunshine.

Even today in most of the districts, the houses face south, with the doors and windows facing the sun. This causes the rooms to be bright, have fresh air, and to be warm in winter and cool in summer. Trees, flowers, and grass are planted around the houses, making the surroundings beautiful, preventing wind and dust, and conditioning the air.

During the Qing dynasty, a famous healthcare expert named Cao Cishan paid great attention to the living surroundings. Although he lived in a city, he created a good micro-environment in which to live. His house faced a garden that he built with a clear pool in it. Around his house, he planted many pine trees so that he could hear the sound of the wind between the trees as if he were living in a valley. He lived until he was greater than ninety years old. In his book, *Lao Lao Neng Yan*, he advocated that old people should plant dozens of flowers and trees of various kinds by themselves. They need not be the exotic or rare types, but they should plant something for every season. This not only beautified the surroundings but also soothed his temperament.

Modern research has indicated that planting trees, flowers, and grass around your home can adjust the temperature, humidity, and the content of carbon dioxide in the air, purify the air, prevent wind and dust, kill bacteria, eliminate noise, and have good effects on the organs of our bodies.

Improving surroundings also includes eliminating the noise and harmful industrial toxic gases so as to create a fine living environment and, thus, promote health and longevity.

Improvement of Cleanliness and Sanitation. Keeping your living surroundings clean is another important measure that prevents illness. China's earliest inscriptions on bones or tortoise shells contain records of general cleaning instructions stating, "When the cock crows for the first time, one should clean the house and sweep the yard." This was written over two thousand years ago and shows that even then great attention was paid to sanitation.

Aside from everyday cleaning and cleaning before the spring festival, people then used red orpiment liquor and the burning of incense as a type of disinfectant.

The ancient Chinese also understood the importance of keeping ditches and irrigation canals open.

CHAPTER 2

Practical Chinese Materia Medica for Healthcare

2.1 Commonly Used Chinese Material Medicines for Healthcare

Chinese material medicines for healthcare are those that can supplement the body with nutrients, enhance the body's functions, strengthen resistance, build up health or promote recovery, and increase longevity. They are also called tonics because of their tonifying properties. Based of their effects and indications, such tonics are classified according to five kinds. They are *qi* tonics, blood tonics, *yang* tonics, *yin* tonics, and other tonics.

2.1.1 *Qi* TONICS

Qi tonics are those drugs that replenish *qi* and eliminate syndromes due to *qi* deficiency.

All life activities, such as growth, development, and metabolism, are dependent on *qi*. The spleen is the source of *qi* and blood, and the lungs dominate the *qi* of the whole body. As a result, the formation and circulation of *qi* in the body depends on whether the spleen and lung function normally. Dysfunction of the spleen and lung due to one cause or another will result in the syndrome known as *qi* deficiency. If you are *qi* deficient, your body will become weak, and symptoms such as fatigue, lassitude, listlessness, poor appetite, languor, and spontaneous sweating will manifest.

Qi tonics can remove or relieve the syndrome of *qi* deficiency and promote recovery. Some *qi* tonics—such as *Ren Shen* (Radix Ginseng), *Da Zao* (Fructus Jujubae), *Feng Huang Jiang* (royal jelly), *Ci Wu Jia* (Radix Acanthopanacis Senticosi), *Yi Tang* (Saccharum Granorum), and *Feng Mi* (Mel)—may play a role in maintaining good health and prolonging life. This is true when any of them is taken in autumn and winter in small dose by the old or by the middle-aged with delicate constitution.

Tonics are chosen according to the symptoms of *qi* deficiency. The syndrome of *qi* deficiency should be treated on the basis of overall analysis of its main and accompanying symptoms. Excessive intake of *qi* tonics must be avoided, or *qi* will be stagnated. The following is a more detailed description of those *qi* tonics named above.

Ren Shen (Radix Ginseng). *Ren Shen* is named according to its original growing area. If it grows in the Jilin province of China, it is called *Jilin Shen*, from Korea, *Gaoli Shen*. The best produced comes from Fusong county in Jilin province of China.

Ren Shen is also named according to the way it is processed. That which is sun-dried is known as *Gan Shen*. When it is soaked in syrup before it is dried, it is called *Tang Shen*. When the herb is steamed and then dried, it is called *Hong Shen*.

Ren Shen has a sweet and a bitter taste and is slightly warm in nature. It is a good tonic in the winter. It has the potency to invigorate primordial *qi*, reinforce the spleen, benefit the lungs, promote the production of body fluid, quench thirst, tranquilize the mind, and help develop intelligence. People who are old or weak may take small doses of *Ren Shen* when they have no appetite and feel tired and sleepy but have difficulty falling asleep. In so doing, their *qi* will be invigorated, their minds tranquilized, their appetite improved, and their bodily strength restored. In clinical practices, *Ren Shen* is often administered to patients whose *qi* is deficient due to prolonged disease, patients in various kinds of shock, and those whose *qi* and *yin* are both deficient. Pharmacological studies have proved that the main active component of *Ren Shen* is ginsenoside. This component can improve the functions of various organs, especially those of the nervous, circulatory, and endocrine systems. It also enhances the immune system and the ability of the body to adapt to its natural environment, thus strengthening the body and contributing to longevity.

Ren Shen is applicable to the syndrome of *qi* deficiency. It is not recommended for those with a strong constitution. It is incompatible with *Li Lu* (*Rhizoma et Radix Veratri*), *Wu Ling Zhi* (*Faeces Trogopterori*), and *Za Jia* (*Spina Gleditsiae*). For oral use, Ren Shen is decocted in water. The usual dosage is 5–10grams. While taking *Ren Shen*, avoid tea and radish.

Xi Yang Shen (Radix Panacis Quinquefolii). *Xi Yang Shen* has a bitter and slightly sweet taste; it is cold in nature and has the potency to invigorate *qi*, nourish *yin*, clear away heat, and promote the production of body fluid. Because it is slow acting, it is very suitable for use with children that have a high fever. It is also used to treat excessive thirst, dehydration due to diarrhea, fever of the deficiency-type, and irritating dry cough due to pulmonary tuberculosis. In addition, it may be used to treat disorders due to the damage of both *qi* and *yin*, regardless of the cause.

Studies have shown that *Xi Yang Shen* contains the active components panasenoside and ginsenoside. These components work together to reduce fever, promote the formation of antibodies, improve the immune function, and strengthen the body.

Xi Yang Shen is decocted in water for oral use. Its usual dosage is 3–6 grams. Be sure not to administer it together with *Li Lu* (Rhizoma et Radix Veratri), nor to parch it on ironwork.

Tai Zi Shen (Radix Pseudostellariae). *Tai Zi Shen* is sweet in taste and neutral in nature. It has a potency similar to that of *Ren Shen*; it invigorates *qi*, promotes the production of body fluid, reinforces the spleen, and tonifies the lung. Because it is a mild and not too greasy tonic, it is often administered to those who have just recovered from illness but remain debilitated, It is also given to those who are old or weak and those who feel listless or have no appetite. In addition, it is often used as a substitute for *Xi Yang Shen* to treat those who have less saliva and feel thirsty when diseases are in the later stages, when *qi* and *yin* have been both consumed, and when the pathogenic factors or diseases have not been cleared away completely.

Tai Zi Shen is known to contain the main active components of saponin, fructose and starch. It is decocted in water for oral use, with the usual dosage being 10–30 grams.

Ci Wu Jia (Radix Acanthopanacis Senticosi). *Ci Wu Jia* is acrid and slightly bitter in taste and warm in nature. It has the potency to replenish *qi* invigorate the spleen, tonify the kidney, tranquilize the mind, expel wind, and remove dampness. It is an important tonic for strengthening the body's resistance and for restoring normal functioning of the body to consolidate the constitution. It is used with good results for senile disorders, menopausal syndrome, primary hypertension, hypotension, paralytic or excitatory impotence, and toxicant poisoning. Furthermore, it is suitable for athletes, divers, and people working at high altitudes.

Ci Wu Jia is known to contain a variety of eleutherosides, organic acids, and ten trace elements as its main active components. Its pharmacological actions include: double regulation of the central nervous system and blood pressure, relief of fatigue, increase in the efficiency of mental and manual labor, enhancement of longevity, improvement of immune function, increase of the body's resistance to harmful factors, stimulation of the sexual and adrenal glands, decrease in blood sugar level, decrease in the growth of tumors, and adjustment of whole body functions.

Ci Wu Jia is decocted in water for oral use or put in other dosage forms when taken. The usual dosage is 9–30 grams.

Dang Shen (Radix Codonopsis). *Dang Shen* comes from the Shangdang district of Shanxi province of China. There are two types, the wild type and the cultivated type. The wild type is named *Ye Tai Dang*, the cultivated, *Lu Dang Shen*. *Dang Shen* is sweet in taste and neutral in nature. It has the potency to promote the production of body fluid, nourish the blood, invigorate the spleen, and replenish *qi*. Its main active components are saponin, protein, and vitamins. It is used as a longevity-promoting tonic, is not toxic, and is also suitable for disorders of *qi* deficiency and various kinds of anemia. For treating those conditions that occur due to the general deficiency of *qi* and weakened body resistance, *Dang Shen* may be administered together with diaphoretic or purgative. This will strengthen the body's resistance and help eliminate pathogenic factors.

Dang Shen has been known to stimulate the central nervous system, relieve fatigue, lower blood pressure, raise blood sugar levels, promote the production of red blood cells and hemoglobin, improve the immune function, and enhance resistance to disease.

Dang Shen is incompatible with *Li Lu* (*Rhizoma et Radix Veratri*). When taking *Dang Shen*, avoid radish and tea. For oral usage, it is decocted in water. The usual dosage is 10–30 grams.

Huang Qi (Radix Astragali). *Huang Qi* is sweet in taste and slightly warm in nature. It has the potency to replenish *qi*, keep *yang-qi* ascending, supplement the defensive-*qi*, consolidate superficial resistance, promote pus discharge and tissue regeneration, and relieve edema. It is a commonly used *qi* tonic suitable for such syndromes as *qi* deficiency of the spleen and lungs, sinking of the *qi* in middle *jiao*, spontaneous sweating due to exterior deficiency. It can also be used to treat such disorders as edema and carbuncles or boils that are slow in healing. Pharmacological researchers have proved that *Huang Qi* mainly contains coumarin, flavone, and saponin as its active components. It plays a role in lowering blood pressure, tonifying the heart, inhibiting bacteria, protecting the liver, relieving the pathogenic changes of the kidney, stimulating the central nervous system, functioning as a sexual hormone, and strengthening the body. It is advisable to prescribe *Huang Qi* in the treatment of gastroptosia, hysteroptosis, proctoptosis, long-standing diarrhea and dysentery, incontinence of urine, and chronic nephritis.

Huang Qi is decocted in water for oral use. The usual dosage is 10–30 grams.

Bai Zhu (Rhizoma Atractylodis Macrocephalae). *Bai Zhu* is bitter and sweet in taste and warm in nature. It is a choice tonic, which is used to replenish *qi*, invigorate the spleen, eliminate dampness, promote diuresis, arrest profuse or spontaneous sweating, and prevent miscarriages. It is often used to treat chronic dyspepsia, chronic nonspecific colitis, edema due to hypofunction of the spleen, nephrogenic edema, alimentary, edema, edema of pregnancy, miscarriage, spontaneous sweating due to general deficiency of *qi*, and chronic rheumatic arthritis. *Bai Zhu* is known to contain atractylol, atractylone, and vitamin A. Pharmacological actions include reducing blood sugar levels, improving blood coagulation, stimulating peristalsis, harmonizing the internal environment with the external, inhibiting cell mutations.

Bai Zhu is decocted in water for oral use. The usual dosage is 5–15 grams.

Gan Cao (Radix Glycyrrhizae). *Gan Cao* is sweet in taste and neutral in nature. It invigorates the spleen, replenishes *qi*, moisturizes the lungs, arrests cough, relieves spasms and pain, and moderates the properties of other drugs. Clinically, it is used in harmonizing the properties of drugs in various kinds of prescriptions. It is also used in treating gastro-duodenal ulcers, infective hepatitis, Addison's disease, bronchial asthma, pulmonary tuberculosis, thrombocytopenic purpura, and thrombotic phlebitis. Research has proved that *Gan Cao* mainly contains glycyrrhizin, glycyrrhetinic acid, liquiritigenin, and liquiritin. It improves the function of the digestive system, acts as a detoxifying agent, lowers fever, relieves cough and asthma, resists inflammation and allergy, reduces cholesterol, and helps the condition atherosclerosis.

Gan Cao is incompatible with *Hai Zao (Sargassum), Da Ji (Radix Knoxiae), Gan Sui (Radix Kansui),* and *Yuan Hua (Flos Genkwa).* It is decocted in water for oral use. The usual dosage is 3–15 grams. Dosages that are larger than recommended can cause edema and elevated blood pressure.

Shan Yao (Rhizoma Dioscoreae). *Shan Yao* is sweet and mild-natured. It is used to supplement *qi*, nourish *yin*, and tonify the spleen, lungs, and kidneys. *Shan Yao* is produced in Xinxiang county, a part of Henan province. The finest quality *Shan Yao* is called *Huai Shan Yao.* Its main active components are saponin, phlegm, choline, glucoprotein, amino acids, vitamin C, and dopamine. Its pharmacological actions include inducing the formation of interferon, enhancing immunological functions, promoting the flow of blood in the coronary arteries and capillaries, relieving coughs and asthma, removing sputum, and strengthening the body.

Shan Yao is a mild tonic for nourishing the spleen and stomach and is used in treating diarrhea due to the hypofunction of the spleen, cough due to the hypofunction of the lungs, diabetes, spermatorrhea, frequent urination, chronic nephritis, and emaciation due to consumption.

Shan Yao is decocted in water for oral use. The usual dosage is 10–30 grams.

Huang Jing (Rhizoma Polygonati). *Huang Jing* is sweet in taste and neutral in nature. It is a longevity-enhancing tonic, and it invigorates the spleen, replenishes *qi*, moisturizes the lungs, and nourishes *yin*. It is often used to treat chronic malnutrition, pulmonary tuberculosis, insufficiency of primordial energy due to a kidney deficiency, and weakness of the spleen and stomach. Furthermore, it can be used as a tonic for building up the health of the old. *Huang Jing* mainly contains nicotinic acid, quinone, phlegm, sugar, and alkaloid. Its pharmacological actions include decreasing blood sugar levels, lowering blood pressure, inhibiting bacteria, resisting tuberculosis, preventing atherosclerosis, increasing the number of T-cells and enhancing their function, prolonging the life of somatic cells, and strengthening the body to retard aging and increase longevity.

Huang Jing is decocted in water for oral use. The usual dosage of the dried herb is 10–20 grams; the dosage of the fresh herb is 30–60 grams.

Da Zao (Fructus Jujubae). *Da Zao* is sweet in taste and warm in nature. It is a longevity-enhancing tonic and is also used to invigorate the spleen, replenish *qi*, nourish the blood, calm the mind, and moderate the properties and tastes of other drugs.

A healthy individual taking a decoction of *Da Zao* will have his or her acquired constitution strengthened. Studies have proved that *Da Zao* mainly contains protein, sugar, organic acids, and vitamins. Its pharmacological actions include increasing the strength of the muscles, protecting the liver, improvement of allergic symptoms, tranquilizing the mind and promoting urination. *Da Zao* is decocted in water for oral use. The usual dosage is 3–12 dates or 10–30 grams.

Yi Tang (Saccharum Granorum). *Yi Tang* is sweet in taste and warm in nature. It is a fine tonic that is used to invigorate the spleen, replenish *qi*, relieve spasms and pain, moisturize the lungs, and arrest coughs. Its indications are gastric ulcer, duodenal bulbar ulcer, chronic gastritis, cough due to the lung deficiency, chronic bronchitis, and pulmonary tuberculosis.

Modern pharmacological research has also proved that *Yi Tang* has the power to strengthen the stomach, moisten the lungs, and arrest coughs.

Yi Tang is dissolved in a decoction and taken 2–3 times daily. The usual dosage is 30–60 grams.

Feng Mi (Mel). *Feng Mi* is sweet in taste and neutral in nature. It reinforces the function of the spleen and stomach, alleviates spasms, moistens the lungs, arrests coughs, and relaxes the bowels. This tonic is suitable for use with ulcerous disorders and chronic hepatitis and for syndromes such as infirmity with age, lack of body fluid during convalescence, constipation due to dry feces, and prolonged cough due to consumption. Applied externally, it may be used to treat the skin for burns and external diseases. When it is taken orally, it is used to detoxify *Chuan Wu (Radix Aconiti), Fu Zi (Radix Aconiti)*. It is often used to help process other Chinese drugs or is an ingredient of other preparations.

Pharmacological studies have proved that *Feng Mi* (with sugar, inorganic salt, enzyme, protein, pigment and pollen grain as its main active principles) has the power to inhibit bacteria and strengthen the body. Elders benefit by taking *Feng Mi* frequently.

Feng Mi is taken after being infused in boiled water, the usual dosage being 15–30 grams.

2.1.2 BLOOD TONICS

Blood tonics are drugs that enrich the blood and improve or eliminate the syndrome of blood deficiency.

The main signs and symptoms of blood deficiency are sallow complexion, pale lips and tongue, giddiness, numbness of the extremities, and palpitations. Blood tonics play an active part in promoting the general circulation of blood and harmonizing the functions of the internal organs, thus slowing down senility.

Most blood tonics are viscous and greasy. Taking too much of any of them will affect your appetite.

E Jiao (Colla Corfi Asini). *E Jiao* originated in Shandong province. *E Jiao* that is produced by the refineries in the Pingyin and Donge counties of Shandong province is the best and most famous in the world.

E Jiao is sweet in taste and neutral in nature. It is used to tonify the blood, arrest bleeding, nourish *yin*, and moisten the lungs. It is also used as an essential tonic used to treat the syndrome of blood deficiency. *E Jiao* has a variety of indications including various kinds of anemia, hemorrhage, and gynecopathy.

Pharmacological experiments have proved that the main components of *E Jiao* include amino acids, calcium, and sulfur. *E Jiao* can raise the number of red blood cells and the amount of hemoglobin, prevent and treat progressive dystrophy, promote calcium equilibrium in the body, improve the immunological function of the body, and elevate blood pressure.

E Jiao is dissolved in boiled water or yellow rice wine or is melted in a decoction before taking. The usual dosage is 5–10 grams.

Dang Gui (Radix Angeticae Sinensis). *Dang Gui* is mainly produced in Min county, located in the southeast portion of Gansu province of China. It is an effective tonic that has a sweet and pungent taste and is warm in nature.

It is used to nourish the blood, promote blood circulation, alleviate pain and moisten the intestines. The chief active components of this herb are sugar, amino acids, inorganic elements, and vitamins. The pharmacological effects include tonifying the heart, dilating coronary arteries, lowering blood pressure and cholesterol levels, relieving atherosclerosis, resisting pernicious anemia, tranquilizing the mind, easing pain, combating bacteria, protecting the liver, and dually-regulating the uterus. Other indications include hypertension, coronary heart disease, cerebral arteriosclerosis, various kinds of anemia, thromboangiitis obliterans, constipation, gynecopathy such as irregular menstruation and all syndromes that are caused due to blood deficiency.

The middle part of the *Dang Gui* root is used to nourish the blood and the tips are used to remove blood stasis. The whole root is used to enrich the blood and promote blood circulation. *Dang Gui* that is processed with liquor will have greater results promoting the flow of the blood.

It should be decocted in water for oral use. The usual dosage is 5–15 grams.

Shu Di Huang (Radix Rehmanniae Praeparata). *Shu Di Huang* is a vegetable tonic used for prolonging life. It is sweet in taste and slightly warm in nature. It nourishes the blood, replenishes *yin*, and invigorates marrow. Its main active components are ß-sitosterol, mannitol, rehmannin, alkaloid, fatty acids, glucose, amino acids, and vitamin A. The pharmacological actions include resisting inflammation, combating bacteria, protecting the liver, inducing diuresis, functioning as a sexual hormone, improving the circulatory system, lowering blood sugar concentration, and preventing leukopenia due to chemotherapy. Indications for the use of *Shu Di Huang* include the syndrome due to blood deficiency. This deficiency is indicated by a pale complexion, dizziness, palpitations, insomnia, irregular menstruation, and abnormal uterine discharge. Other indications include the syndrome due to *yin* deficiency of the liver and kidney, diabetes, infective hepatitis, rheumatic arthritis, and rheumatoid arthritis.

Shu Di Huang is decocted for oral dose; the usual dosage is 10–30 grams.

He Shou Wu (Radix Polygoni Multiflori). *He Shou Wu* is bitter, sweet, and astringent in taste and slightly warm in nature. It is a tonic that is used to nourish the blood, replenish the vital essence, prevent the attack of malaria, relax the bowels, strengthen the bones and tendons, keep hair black, and promote longevity. It is also used to treat the syndrome due to *yin* and blood deficiency, early-graying of hair, prolonged malaria, pyogenic infections, skin and external diseases, constipation, hypertension, coronary heart disease and elevated cholesterol levels.

Its active components include chrysophanol, emodin, rhein, phscion, and lecithin. *He Shou Wu* exerts the following pharmacological actions: reducing blood-fat, alleviating atherosclerosis, functioning as adrenocortical hormone, strengthening the heart, relieving constipation, and inhibiting bacteria.

He Shou Wu is decocted in water for oral use. The usual dosage is 10–30 grams. *Zhi* (prepared) *He Shou Wu* is prescribed to tonify the blood and vital essence.

Bai Shao (Radix Paeoniae Alba). *Bai Shao* is bitter and sour in taste and slightly cold in nature. As a commonly used blood tonic, it is used to nourish the blood, calm the liver, arrest pain, and suppress hyperactivity of the liver-*yang*. It is often administered to treat spasms of the limbs and irregular menstruation due to blood deficiency, abdominal pain due to the stagnation of the liver-*qi*, spontaneous perspiration and night sweating due to blood deficiency and hyperactivity of the liver, ulcerative diseases, and gastroenteritis.

Modern pharmacological studies have proven that *Bai Shao* mainly contains paeoniflorin, paeonol, ß-sitosterol, volatile oil, resin, fatty oil, sugar, starch, phlegm, and protein. It plays a role in anti-inflammation, ulcer-prevention, anti-spasm, anti-bacteria, sedation, analgesia, dilation of coronary arteries, enhancement of body resistance, anti-perspiration, and diuresis.

Bai Shao is decocted in water for oral use. The usual dosage is 10–30 grams.

Long Yan Rou (Arillus Longan). *Long Yan* (longan) is an appetizing fruit used in the making of *Long Yan Rou*, which is a choice tonic for those old in age to build up their health and prolong their lives. *Long Yan Rou* is sweet in taste and warm in nature. It has the power to tonify the heart and spleen and replenish *qi* and blood. It is often prescribed to treat neurosism due to the deficiency of both the heart and spleen, the syndrome due to *qi* and blood deficiency, chronic bleeding due to general deficiency, profuse menstruation due to blood deficiency, postpartum edema, pulmonary tuberculosis, hypertension and coronary heart disease.

Studies have shown that the main active components of *Long Yan Rou* are saponin, fatty oil, fatty acid, sugar, vitamins, and choline. The pharmacological actions include anti-bacterial, anti-cancer, sedation, lowering of blood-fat, enrichment of coronary blood flow, and enhancement of constitution.

Long Yan Rou is made into a decoction or liquid extract, soaked in liquor, or made into pills, for oral use. The usual dosage is 10–15 grams.

Sang Shen (Fructus Mori). *Sang Shen* is an effective tonic that is used for nourishing the blood and *yin*. It is able to replenish *yin* and the blood, promote the production of body fluid, and moisturize the intestines. This tonic is used for the treatment of the syndrome caused by blood and *yin* deficiency. This syndrome is marked by dizziness, tinnitus, insomnia, premature-graying of hair, and constipation, as well as diabetes, hypertension, artheriosclerosis, various kinds of anemia, and neurosism. Studies prove that *Sang Shen* mainly contains rutin, anthocyanin, carotin, vitamins, nicotinic acid, sugar, and fatty oils. It contributes to the increase of number and function of T-cells, the improvement of the immunologic function, good health, and long life.

Sang Shen is eaten raw or as a decoction or liquid extract or is soaked in liquor for oral dosage. The usual dose is 10–15 grams.

2.1.3 YANG TONICS

Yang tonics are those drugs that support the *yang-qi* of the body and relieve or eliminate syndromes due to *yang* deficiency.

Yang deficiency includes the deficiency of the heart-*yang*, the spleen-*yang*, and the kidney-*yang*. Of the three kinds of *yang-qi*, the most important is the kidney-*yang*, upon which the *zang* and *fu* organs depend in order to be warmed and to give full play to their physiological function. For this reason deficiency of kidney-*yang* is closely related to various syndromes caused by *yang* deficiency. The syndrome of kidney-*yang* deficiency manifests as aversion to cold, cold limbs, weakness and soreness of the loins and knees, weak constitution, listlessness, lack of sexual desire, and excessive night urine.

Yang tonics have the potency to alleviate or remove the syndrome of *yang* deficiency and retard senility because they have the power to tonify the kidney-*yang*, nourish the marrow and strengthen the bones and tendons. Modern pharmacological researches have proven that *Yang* tonics can regulate adrenocortical function, adjust energy metabolism, improve gonadal function, and promote growth and development and enhance the body's resistance.

Healthy persons should be careful when taking *yang* tonics because most of them are warm and dry in nature.

Lu Rong (Cornu Cervi Pantotrichum). As one of the rare Chinese drugs, *Lu Rong* is sweet and salty in taste and warm in nature. It is an important and powerful tonic, which has the potency to invigorate kidney-*yang*, replenish the vital essence and blood, and strengthen the bones and tendons. It is often administered to treat impotence, spermatorrhea, infertility, children's maldevelopment, severe anemia, rheumatic heart disease, neurosism, and unhealing ulcers.

The active components of *Lu Rong* include pantocrine, calcium phosphate, calcium carbonate, colloids, protein, phosphorus, magnesium, cholesterol, and vitamin A.

The pharmacological effects of this tonic function like a powerful androgenic hormone. Such effects include promotion of protein synthesis, raising the number of white blood cells, enhancing the body's functions, promoting growth and development, stimulating rapid healing of fractures and ulcers, strengthening the heart, inducing diuresis, increasing the womb's strength to expand and contract, improving metabolic energy.

Lu Rong is ground into powder and taken with boiled water. The usual dosage is 1–3 grams, divided into thirds and taken in intervals.

Ge Jie (Gecko). *Ge Jie* is an animal *yang* tonic produced mainly in Guangxi province of China. It is salty in taste and neutral in nature. It is used to invigorate lung-*qi*, tonify the kidney-*yang*, relieve asthma and cough, and replenish the vital essence and blood. It is often administered to treat prolonged cough with blood due to pulmonary tuberculosis, bronchial asthma, pulmonary emphysema, impotence, frequent urination, and neurosis.

Studies have shown that *Ge Jie* contains protein, fat, and starch and can (directly or indirectly) stimulate the sex glands, enhance the body's functions, and promote growth and development.

Ge Jie is decocted in water or ground into powder and soaked in liquor for oral use. If decocted in water, the usual dosage is 3–7 grams. If it is ground into powder, 1–2 grams of powder is taken with boiled water three times a day. If it is soaked in liquor, 1–2 pairs of *Ge Jie* (geckoes) are soaked each time and the medicated liquor is drunk according to the doctor's orders.

Ba Ji Tian (Radix Morindae Officinalis). *Ba Ji Tian* is acrid and sweet in taste and slightly warm in nature. It is an essential drug for tonifying the kidney. This tonic is used to reinforce the kidney, support *yang*, expel wind, remove dampness, and prolong life. Indications for this tonic are impotence, incontinence of urine, frequent urination, infertility, and irregular menstruation. Its main active elements are morindin, vitamin C, sugar, and resin. Its pharmacological effects strengthen the heart, dilate the coronary arteries, lower blood pressure, combat bacteria, remove phlegm, relieve cough and asthma, enhance the immunologic function, and prevent leukopenia.

Ba Ji Tian is decocted in water for oral use. The usual dosage is 10–15 grams.

Du Zhong (Cortex Eucommiae). *Du Zhong* is sweet to taste and warm in nature. It is used to tonify the liver and kidneys, strengthen the bones and tendons, and prevent abortion. It is a highly effective drug for strengthening the body and prolonging life, and it is suitable for the treatment deficiency of the liver and kidneys, weakness and soreness of the loins and knees, hypertension, sequel of poliomyelitis, threatened abortion, and frequent miscarriages. *Du Zhong* contains mainly gutta-percha, resin, glucoprotein, organic acids, and vitamin C. Its use plays an important part in lowering blood pressure, inducing diuresis, reducing cholesterol, relaxing the womb, and tranquilizing the mind by restraining the central nervous system.

Du Zhong is decocted in water for oral use. Stir-fried *Du Zhong* is more effective.

Dong Chong Xia Cao (Cordyceps). *Dong Chong Xia Cao* is a famous and precious tonic. It is sweet to taste and warm in nature. It nourishes the kidneys, tonifies the lungs, arrests bleeding, resolves phlegm, restores *qi*, consolidates constitution, and enhances longevity. Its use is best suited to those who are weak and susceptible to cold and those who are old and need to consolidate their constitutions through strengthening their body resistance. It is also used in the treatment of anemia, impotence, spermatorrhea, weakness and soreness of the loins and knees, asthma, and cough with blood due to pulmonary tuberculosis.

Dong Chong Xia Cao mainly contains the following active elements: cordycepic acid, cordycepin, protein, fat, vitamin B, amino acids, cordypolysaccharide, uracil, and adenosine. Its pharmacological effects include tranquilizing the mind, relieving spasm, resisting inflammation, combating bacteria, removing phlegm, preventing cough, alleviating asthma, resisting the development of neoplasm, lowering blood pressure, dilating the coronary arteries, reducing blood-fat, and enhancing hypoxia tolerance under ordinary pressure.

The usual dose of *Dong Chong Xia Cao* is 5–10 grams. It is boiled in water and taken orally as a decoction, made into pill or powder form to be taken with boiled water, or stewed and eaten with chicken, duck, or fish.

Zi He Che (Placenta Hominis). *Zi He Che* refers to a woman's placenta, which is an excellent tonic for warming the kidney and strengthening *yang*. It is sweet and salty in taste and warm in property. It is used in replenishing vital essence, nourishing blood and invigorating *qi*. It is used to build up the constitutions of those that are old; prevent hepatitis and influenza; and treat infertility, impotence, and spermatorrhea due to the deficiency of kidney-*qi*. This tonic is also used to treat the vital essence and blood, as well as emaciation, lassitude, sallow complexion and inability to lactate after giving birth due to deficiency of both *qi* and blood; it is also used to treat asthma due to deficiency of both the lungs and kidney.

Zi He Che has been found to contain amino acids, immune factors, and hormones. It also plays a part in promoting the development of the sex glands and reproductive organs, preventing leukopenia, activating the immune system, stimulating the body to function fully and bringing about an advance in the growth and development of the body.

Zi He Che is ground into power and put into capsules to be taken with boiled water. The usual dose is 1.5–3.0 grams, taken 2–3 times daily. Alternatively, a whole or half *Zi He Che* may be boiled in water and eaten together with the broth.

Tu Si Zi (Semen Cuscutae). *Tu Si Zi* is acrid and sweet in taste and neutral in nature. It can invigorate *yang*, replenish *yin*, control spontaneous emission, arrest diuresis, relieve diarrhea, and improve acuity of sight. This tonic is commonly used for tonifying the kidney-*yang* and enhancing longevity, and it is suitable for the treatment of weakness and soreness of the loins and knees due to kidney deficiency. Additionally it is used to treat frequent urination, spermatorrhea, habitual abortion, hypertension, hypoposia, and diabetes.

Pharmacological research has found that the main ingredients of *Tu Si Zi* include resinous glucoside, ß-sitosterol, sugar, amylase, and vitamin A.

Use of this tonic will lower blood pressure, strengthen the heart, inhibit bacteria, stimulate the uterus, regulate immune function, enhance the function of the whole body, and adjust and raise the metabolic function of the body.

Tu Si Zi is decocted in water for oral dosage. The usual dosage is 10–15 grams.

Hu Tao Ren (Semen Juglandis). *Hu Tao Ren* is a popular food with a highly nutritive value. It is a good tonic for the old and the debilitated. *Hu Tao Ren* is sweet in taste and warm in property. It is used to tonify the kidney, warm the lungs, moisturize the intestines and consolidate the constitution. It is used to treat chronic asthmatic bronchitis, lumbago due to kidney deficiency, weak legs, habitual constipation, and urinary calculus.

Hu Tao Ren contains fatty oil, protein, carbohydrate, calcium, phosphorus, iron, carotin, and ovoflavin. *Hu Tao Ren* helps to lower blood pressure and aids in controlling inflammation.

Hu Tao Ren is decocted in water for oral use or eaten raw. The usual dosage is 10–30 grams.

Yang Qi Shi (Actinolitum). *Yang Qi Shi* contains magnesium and calcium silicate as its components. It is salty to taste and slightly warm in nature. *Yang Qi Shi* can warm the kidney and invigorate *yang*. It is a mineral tonic applicable to the treatment of such disorders as cold penis and impotence due to the deficiency of the kidney-*yang*, cold uterus, women's pruritus genitalium of dampness-type, and cold loins and knees as well.

Yang Qi Shi is processed into pills or powder and taken orally with boiled water. The usual dosage is 3–6 grams. Prolonged administration of it is avoided.

Bu Gu Zhi (Fructus Psoraleae). *Bu Gu Zhi* is bitter and acrid in taste and very warm in nature. This tonic can invigorate the kidney-*yang*, control spontaneous emission, warm the spleen, and treat diarrhea. It is a commonly used kidney-*yang* tonic suitable for the treatment of impotence, spermatorrhea, enuresis, frequent urination, cold-pain of the loins and knees, diarrhea due to *yang* deficiency, endometrorrhagia, psoriasis, and vitiligo.

Bu Gu Zhi contains saponin, resin, organic acids, psoralen, psoralidine, and ispsoralene.

Pharmacologically it functions like a female sex hormone, it also dilates the coronary arteries, strengthens the heart, tranquilizes the mind, relieves spasms, stimulates the smooth muscles, combats bacteria, and promotes the formation of pigment cells of the skin and the immunologic function of the body.

Bu Gu Zhi is decocted in water for oral dosage, but it should not be taken by pregnant women. The usual dosage is 5–10 grams.

Yin Yang Huo (Herba Epimedii). *Yin Yang Huo* is acrid and sweet in taste and warm in nature. It can invigorate the kidney-*yang*, expel wind, and remove dampness. It is a highly potent tonic for healthcare and is used in the treatment of impotence, spermatorrhea, frequent urination, weakness and soreness of lions and knees, rheumalalgia, numbness of the limbs, poliomyelitis, women's climacteric hypertension, coronary heart disease, and chronic bronchitis.

Pharmacological show that *Yin Yang Huo* contains icariine, glucoside of flavone, sterol, volatile oils, and vitamin E as its main active components. It has male sex hormone-like actions and plays a part in lowering blood pressure, strengthening the heart, dilating the coronary arteries, inhibiting bacteria, combating viruses, reducing blood sugar levels, regulating the immunologic function, and enhancing adrenocortical functions.

2.1.4 *YIN* TONICS

Yin tonics are all the Chinese drugs that nourish *yin*, promote the production of body fluids, eliminate dryness, and improve or eliminate *yin* deficiency. *Yin* deficiency includes the deficiency of the *jung-yin*, the stomach-*yin*, the liver-*yin*, and the kidney-*yin*. The syndrome of *yin* deficiency is often seen in those that are old and those that are in the advanced stages of febrile disease or in the course of a number of chronic diseases. In general, *yin* deficiency manifests as dry mouth, dry cough with little sputum, afternoon fever, night sweating, irritability, insomnia, spermatorrhea, dizziness, and dry sensation of the eyes. *Yin* tonics promote the production of body fluids, moisturizing dryness and strengthening the body by way of improving sucroclastic metabolism to return hyperfunctional energy metabolism to normal, enhancing immunologic function, and regulating the body fluid metabolism.

Yin tonics are contraindicated in such cases where syndromes of weakness of the spleen and stomach, internal stagnation of phlegm and dampness, or abdominal distension and loose stools are present. This occurs because most *yin* tonics are sweet in taste and cold, viscid, and greasy in nature.

Sha Shen (Radix Adenophorae or Radix Glehnia). There are two types of *Sha Shen: Nan Sha Shen (Radix Adenophorae)* and *Bei Sha Shen (Radix Glehnia)*. The term *Sha Shen* generally refers to *Nan Sha Shen (Radix Adenophorae)*. Both of them are sweet in taste and slightly cold in nature. They are used to clear away lung-heat, nourish *yin*, replenish the stomach, and promote the production of body fluid. They are nutritious tonics and are also used to treat dry cough with little sputum caused by the lung-*yin* deficiency due to the lung-heat, cough with blood due to pulmonary tuberculosis, dry mouth and tongue, and poor appetite due to excess body fluid caused by febrile diseases. *Sha Shen* can also be used to reduce fever, remove phlegm and ease pain.

Pharmacological studies show that *Sha Shen* contains saponin, volatile oils, triterpenoid acid, stigmasterol, ß-sitosterol, and alkaloids.

Sha Shen is decocted in water for oral use. The usual dosage, if dried, is 10–15 grams and 15–30 grams, if fresh. This tonic can be used with *Li Lu* (Rhizoma et Radix Veratri).

Tian Dong (Radix Asparagi). *Tian Dong* is a tonic that is used for strengthening the bones, building up health, delaying senility, and prolonging life. It is sweet and bitter in taste and greatly cold in nature. *Tian Dong* can remove heat from the lungs, replenish *yin,* and moisten dryness. It is administered to treat the following disorders: consumption of *yin* due to febrile diseases, dry cough due to lung deficiency, senile chronic bronchitis, pulmonary tuberculosis, whooping cough, mammary tumors, constipation, and spermatorrhea.

Tian Dong contains mainly 19 kinds of amino acids such as glutamic acid and asparagine, glucose, and steroid saponin. Its pharmacological actions include relieving cough, removing phlegm, combating bacteria, restraining the growth of tumors, improving the function of the heart and lungs, enhancing the ability of the body to adapt to the environment, and decreasing the mutation of body cells.

Tian Dong is decocted in water for oral use. The usual dosage is 10–15 grams.

Shi Hu (Herba Dendrobii). *Shi Hu* is sweet in taste and slightly cold in property. It can nourish the stomach, promote the production of body fluids, replenish *yin* and remove heat.

Because it is a commonly used tonic for nourishing the stomach-*yin*, it is administered to treat disorders that damage body fluid due to febrile disease. It is also used to treat deficiency of stomach-*yin*, consumption of body fluid due to the deficiency of *yin*, persistent fever of *yin* deficiency-type, chronic gastritis, and diabetes.

Shi Hu mainly contains dendrobine, phlegm, and nobilonine. Its actions include reducing fever, easing pain, promoting digestion,

strengthening the heart, lowering blood pressure, preventing leukopenia, enhancing the immunologic function of the body, improving the
metabolism within the body, and regulating the balance of body fluid.

Shi Hu is decocted in water for oral use. If it is administered as an
ingredient of a prescription, it must be the first to be decocted. The
usual dose is 6–15 grams of the dried or 15–30 grams of the fresh.

Mai Dong (Radix Ophiopogonis). *Mai Dong* is sweet and slightly
bitter in taste and a little cold in nature. It can remove dryness from the
lungs, nourish *yin*, reinforce the stomach, promote the production of
body fluid, clear away heat from the heart, and ease mental anxiety. *Mai
Dong* is a tonic that is used for preventing senility and promising
longevity. It is suitable to treat such disorders as dry cough due to lung-
dryness, deficiency of stomach-*yin*, irritability, insomnia, constipation
due to intestinal dryness, expectoration of blood, apostaxis, chronic
pharyngitis, and coronary heart disease.

Mai Dong has been found to contain steroid saponins, ß-sitosterol,
amino acids, glucose, and a vitamin A-like substance. Use of *Mai Dong*
helps improve the function of the cardiovascular system. It also
enhances the ability of the body to adapt to the environment, stop
mutation of body cells, and combat bacteria.

Mai Dong is decocted in water for oral use. The usual dosage is
10–15 grams.

Yu Zhu (Rhizonia Polygonati Odorati). *Yu Zhu* is sweet in taste
and neutral in nature. It can replenish *yin*, remove heat from the lungs,
promote the production of body fluids, and nourish the stomach. It is
weak in potency and non-greasy in nature, so it is a good tonic for the
elderly. *Yu Zhu* is used for treatment of *yin* damage of the spleen and
stomach, heart failure, coronary heart disease, pulmonary tuberculosis,
and diabetes.

Yu Zhu contains the active elements, convallamarin, cofivallarin,
kaempferitrin, quercitrin, vitamin A, and nicotinic acid.

Yu Zhu has a broad spectrum of pharmacological effects, such as
strengthening the heart, dilating the coronary arteries, reducing blood
sugar concentration, combating bacteria, working like adrenocortical
hormone, enhancing the immunologic function of the body, and
improving the function of the heart and lungs. *Yu Zhu* also helps the
body adapt to the environment and improves the function of islet cells
and vasomotor centers.

Yu Zhu is decocted in water for oral use. The usual dosage is 10–15
grams.

Bai He (Bulbus Lilli). *Bai He* is sweet in taste and slightly cold in
nature. It is used to moisten the lungs, to arrest coughs, and clear away

heart-fire to tranquilize the mind. *Bai He* is a commonly used *yin* tonic and is used in the prevention of senility and for longevity as well. It is also applicable to the treatment of cough due to lung-heat, fidgeting of deficiency-type, insomnia or heavy dreaming, chronic nephritis, pulmonary tuberculosis, hypertension, bronchial asthma and chronic bronchitis.

Pharmacological studies prove that *Bai He* contains colchicine, starch, protein, fat, sugar, calcium, phosphorus, and iron.

Bai He removes phlegm, arrests cough, relieves asthma, enhances immunologic function, improves the function of the heart and lungs, and prevents leukopenia.

Bai He can be decocted in water for oral use or taken in gruel or a vegetable dish. The usual dosage of the dried is 10–30 grams, and that of the fresh, 30–50 grams.

Gou Qi Zi (Fructus Lycii). *Gou Qi Zi* is sweet in taste and neutral in nature. It can nourish the liver and kidneys, improve acuity of sight and moisten the lungs. *Gou Qi Zi* is a good tonic for replenishing kidney *yin*, preventing diseases, and prolonging life. This tonic is used for treating *yin* deficiency of the liver and kidney, cough due to *Yin* deficiency, chronic nephritis, chronic hepatitis, cirrhosis, diabetes, and tumors.

The active components of *Gou Qi Zi* are betaine, carotene, zeaxanthin, nicotinic acid, and vitamins.

Its pharmacological actions include: lowering blood sugar and blood-fat levels, lowering blood pressure, enhancing the immunologic function, protecting the liver, and improving leukopenia.

Gou Qi Zi is decocted in water for oral use. The usual dosage is 5–10 grams.

Nü Zhen Zi (Fructus Ligustri Lucidi). *Nü Zhen Zi* is sweet and bitter in taste and cool in nature. It can tonify and nourish the liver and kidney, remove heat, and improve vision. This tonic is commonly used to prevent senility, retard aging, and enhance longevity.

Nü Zhen Zi contains triterpenoid, oleanolic acid, mannitol, glucose, oleic acid, linoleic acid, ligustrin, and fatty acids. Such components work together to play an active part in strengthening the heart, inducing diuresis, protecting the liver, inhibiting bacteria, increasing the number of white blood cells, reducing blood-fat, and enhancing the immunologic function of the body.

Nü Zhen Zi is used to treat the following disorders: *yin* deficiency of the liver and kidney, dizziness, weakness and soreness of the loins and knees, early-graying of hair, blurred vision, chronic nephritis, chronic hepatitis, coronary heart disease, central choroido-retinitis, and leukopenia.

Nü Zhen Zi is decocted in water for oral use. The usual dosage is 10–15 grams.

Hei Zhi Ma (Semen Sesami Nigram). *Hei Zhi Ma* is sweet in taste and neutral in nature. It can replenish vital essence and blood, moisten dryness, and relieve constipation.

Pharmacological studies show that *Hei Zhi Ma* contains protein, fatty oil, sugar, fibrin, calcium, phosphorus, iron, vitamins B12 and E, sesamin, and sesamol. These active components help prevent senility and lower blood pressure, blood sugar, and blood-fat levels. It also helps relax the bowels. This tonic is used to treat hypertension, coronary heart disease, arteriosclerosis, neurosis, constipation due to intestinal dryness, *yin* deficiency of the liver and kidneys, dizziness, early-graying of hair, anemia, and agalactosia.

Hei Zhi Ma is decocted in water for oral dose or stir-baked and eaten as a cooked food. The usual dosage is 10–30 grams.

Bie (Trionycis). *Bie* refers is a fresh-water turtle. The flesh of it is sweet in taste and neutral in nature. The shell is salty and cold. *Bie* is an effective tonic for replenishing the vital essence and nourishing the blood. If it is used for its nourishing action, the flesh is best used.

Modern research shows that *Bie* contains mainly protein, fat, carbohydrates, calcium, phosphorus, iron, vitamin, animal gum, keratin, and iodine. It can play an important role in nourishing the body and building up one's health.

Bie can nourish *yin*, suppress hyperactive *yang*, and remove heat from the blood. It can be used to treat the following disorders: *yin* deficiency of the liver and kidney, copos, hectic fever, night sweats, wind stirring due to *yin* deficiency, and hypertension.

One *Bie* is stewed and eaten each time. Alternatively, 10–13 grams of its shell is decocted in water for oral use.

Yin Er (Tremella). *Yin Er* is sweet, tasteless, and mild-natured. It can nourish *yin*, moisten the lungs, and replenish *qi* and blood. As a rare tonic, it may be used to treat hemoptysis due to pulmonary tuberculosis, hypertension, arteriosclerosis, leukopenia, cancer, and general debility due to chronic diseases. Use of this tonic can benefit both young and old persons.

Studies show that the main active elements of *Yin Er* are protein, gummy substance, enzyme, polysaccharides, inorganic salts, and vitamin B.

Pharmacological effects include: enhancing the immunologic function, activating the hematopoietic function, promoting the synthesis of protein and nucleic acid, resisting tumors, and improving pathogenic changes of the respiratory system.

Yin Er is stewed or cooked into thick soup with other food and eaten. The usual dosage is 3–10 grams.

2.1.5 OTHER CHINESE MEDICINES FOR HEALTHCARE

The following Chinese medicines are not classified as tonics according Chinese Materia Medica, but their tonifying actions may be used treat debility, prevent diseases, and prolong life.

With the development of modern pharmacological research, the healthcare functions of many Chinese medicines are continually discovered. The following Chinese medicines are perfectly edible and have few side or toxic effects.

Suan Zao Ren (Semen Ziziphi Spinosae). *Suan Zao Ren* is sweet and mild-natured. It can nourish the heart, ease the mind, and arrest sweating.

Traditionally, it has been only regarded as a sedative. However, modern pharmacological studies have shown that *Suan Zao Ren* is not only a sedative but can be used to ease pain, relieve spasms, prevent convulsions, reduce fever, and lower blood pressure. Additionally, *Suan Zao Ren* is used to improve the function of the cardiovascular and immune systems, stimulate the uterus, arrest shock, alleviate local edema, and invigorate the body. As a result, it is often used as a tonic for older persons.

The main active elements of *Suan Zao Ren* are jujubogenin, sterol, triterpenoid, a high proportion of vegetable oil, vitamin C, and protein.

Suan Zao Ren is decocted in water for oral dose or is eaten raw. It can also be taken in other dosage forms or nutriments such as wine or nonalcoholic beverages. The usual dosage is 6–15 grams.

Shan Zha (Fructus Crataegi). *Shan Zha* is sour and sweet in taste and slightly warm in nature. It can help promote digestion and eliminate blood stasis. It is not only a nutritious and tasty fruit but also a good tonic for the elderly and those suffering with hypertension or coronary heart disease.

Shan Zha contains mainly triterpenes, flavonoid, ß-sitosterol, stearic acid, vitamin C, and carotene. It has the ability to lower blood-fat levels, increase blood flow in the arteries, and prevent arrhythmia. Additionally, its long-term effects include strengthening the heart, inhibiting bacteria, and promoting digestion.

Shan Zha is decocted in water for oral use, eaten raw, or taken in the form of cake, jam, juice, extract, or wine. The usual dosage of the dried is 6–15 grams and of the fresh is 30–50 grams.

Lian Zi (Semen Nelumbinis). *Lian Zi* is sweet and sour in taste and neutral in nature. It can invigorate the spleen to treat diarrhea, tonify the kidney to arrest spontaneous emissions, and nourish the heart to calm the mind. It is traditionally used as an astringent to treat the following disorders: spontaneous emissions, spermatorrhea, frequent urination due to kidney deficiency, prolonged diarrhea due to spleen deficiency, palpitations, restlessness of deficiency-type, and insomnia.

It is known that the main active elements of *Lian Zi* are starch, melitose, protein, fat, carbohydrate, calcium, phosphorus, and iron.

Lian Zi is often used in treating tumors and lowering blood pressure.

Lian Zi is decocted in water for oral use, eaten in a gruel or thick soup, or taken in other dosage forms. The usual dosage is 6–15 grams.

Ling Zhi (Ganoderma Lucidum seu Japonicum). *Ling Zhi* is tasteless and slightly bitter and warm-natured. It can tranquilize the mind and invigorate the spleen and stomach. It is a rare drug, and it has the power to consolidate the constitution by strengthening the body's resistance and restoring the body's normal function. *Ling Zhi* is used to treat angina pectoris due to coronary heart disease, infectious hepatitis, leukopenia, neurosism, and anemia.

It is known that *Ling Zhi* contains mainly alkaloids, peptides, sugar, sterol, triterpenes, volatile oil, resin, 13 kinds of inorganic elements, and 15 different amino acids.

Its pharmacological actions include: strengthening the heart, dilating coronary arteries, preventing atherogenesis, relieving cough, removing phlegm, alleviating asthma, inhibiting bacteria, enhancing the immunologic functions, protecting the liver, tranquilizing the body, easing pain, resisting cancer and activating hematopoietic system.

For oral use, 1.5–3.0 grams of *Ling Zhi* is decocted in water. If it is ground into a powder and swallowed with boiled water then 0.9–1.5 grams is used. *Ling Zhi* may also be soaked in and taken with liquor.

Fu Ling (Poria). *Fu Ling* is sweet, tasteless, and mild-natured. It can promote water metabolism, remove dampness, strengthen the spleen and stomach, and ease mental stress.

Fu Ling contains pachymic acid, P-pachman, choline, protein, fat, ergosterin, kalium, natrium, and lecithin. As one of the more commonly used Chinese medicinal herbs, *Fu Ling* is a nutritious tonic that is used for healthcare and boosting longevity. It is appropriate for the treatment of edema, difficult urination, deficiency of the spleen and stomach, chronic diarrhea, palpitations, insomnia, and Meniere's disease.

The pharmacological actions of *Fu Ling* include inducing diuresis, tranquilizing the body, inhibition of bacterial growth, resisting tumor growth, strengthening the heart, reducing blood sugar levels, improving the function of the digestive system and enhancing the immunological function.

Fu Ling is decocted in water for oral use, prepared into pills or powder, or taken in gruel or cake. The usual dosage is 10–15 grams.

Yi Yi Ren (Semen Coicis). *Yi Yi Ren* is sweet, tasteless, and slightly cold-natured. It can promote water metabolism, remove dampness, and strengthen the spleen. It also relieves stagnation-syndrome of *qi* and blood and clears away heat and discharge.

Yi Yi Ren is administered in the treatment of urinary difficulty, edema, diarrhea due to spleen deficiency, rheumatic arthritis, pulmonary abscess, pulmonary tuberculosis, and cancer. Furthermore, *Yi Yi Ren* may be used as a tonic for people that are old and infirm, especially with stiff limbs.

Modern research has shown that the main active components of *Yi Yi Ren* are protein, fat, carbohydrate, vitamin B, coixol, and coixenolide.

These active ingredients reduce fever, ease pain, strengthen the heart, resist tumors, and improve the function of the respiratory system.

Yi Yi Ren is decocted in water for oral dose or eaten in a gruel. The usual dosage is 10–30 grams.

Qian Shi (Semen Euryales). *Qian Shi* is sweet, sour, and mild-natured. It can replenish the kidneys, check spontaneous emissions, invigorate the spleen, remove dampness and treat diarrhea.

Its main active elements are protein; starch; sugar; fat; vitamins B1, B12, and C; nicotinic acid; carotene; calcium; phosphorus; and iron.

Qian Shi is an excellent tonic for curing diseases and Prolonging life. *Qian Shi* is easy to digest and is suitable for the treatment of the following: prolonged diarrhea due to spleen deficiency, spontaneous emission due to kidney deficiency, incontinence of urine, and leukorrhagia.

Qian Shi is decocted in water for oral dose or eaten in gruel. The usual dosage is 10–15 grams.

Xiang Gu (Lentinus Edodes). *Xiang Gu* is sweet and mild-natured. It has the potency to restore *qi*, strengthen the stomach, and promote the eruption of rashes. It is also used to treat poor appetites, vomitting, diarrhea, lassitude, dribbling urination, turbid urine, pox or measles, cancer, hyperlipernia, rickets, and anemia.

Pharmacological studies have shown that the main active elements in *Xiang Gu* are protein, fats, carbohydrates, vitamins, calcium, phosphorus, iron, and nicotinic acid.

Xiang Gu is used to resist tumors, reduce blood-fat, enhance the immunologic function, and prevent rickets. Recently, people have become more aware of the nutritive and healthcare value of *Xiang Gu* and have used it as an effective tonic for curing disease and prolonging life.

Xiang Gu is decocted in water for oral use, or it is stewed with pork, chicken, or fish. The usual dosage is 6–9 grams.

Mu Er (Auricularia). *Mu Er* is sweet in taste and neutral in nature. It has the potency to invigorate *Qi*, remove pathogenic heat from the blood, and arrest bleeding. It is also used to treat hypertension, coronary heart disease, and various kinds of hemorrhages.

Studies have shown that *Mu Er* contains protein, sugar, lipid, sterol, inorganic salt and vitamins as its main active composition.

The pharmacological functions of *Mu Er* include hemostasis, prevention and treatment of atherosclerosis, and activation of the body and mind. It can also retard the onset of senility. It is not only a suitable food for the dinner table, but it is also a good tonic for preventing diseases, protecting health, and enhancing longevity.

Mu Er is cooked and eaten as a dish or in a thick soup. The usual dosage is 15–30 grams.

Ju Hua (Flos Chrysanthemi). *Ju Hua* is sweet, bitter, and cool-natured. It can expel wind, clear away heat, calm the liver, improve vision, subdue inflammation, and expel toxic substances. *Ju Hua* has been used as an exterior-syndrome-relieving drug to treat wind-heat syndrome due to exopathogens, furuncles, carbuncles, and swelling. Recently, it has been used to treat coronary heart disease and hypertension.

Research shows that the main active principles of *Ju Hua* are volatile oils, chrysanthmin, choline, amino acids, vitamins, adenine, and trace elements.

The pharmacological actions of *Ju Hua* include: improving the function of the cardiovascular system, preventing thrombosis, preventing and treating cardiovascular diseases, reducing fever, tranquilizing the mind, inhibiting bacteria, combating virus, and retarding the onset of senility, and enhancing longevity.

Ju Hua is decocted in water or soaked in liquor and taken orally. Alternatively, it may be infused in boiling water and taken as tea. The usual dosage is 6–9 grams.

Dan Shen (Radix Salviae Miltiorrhizae). *Dan Shen* is bitter and slightly cold in nature. It is used to cool and nourish the blood, remove blood stasis, promote the circulation of the blood, heal the skin and tranquilize the mind. It is also used as a blood-flow-promoting drug to treat abdominal pain due to blood stasis, abdominal masses, irregular

61

menstruation, amenorrhea due to blood stagnation, skin and external disorders and the syndrome due to the invasion of the blood system by pathogenic heat. Recently, *Dan Shen* has been used effectively in the treatment of coronary heart disease, thromboangiitis obliterans, chronic hepatitis, hepatosplenomegaly, and infantile pneumonia.

Pharmacological studies have shown that the main active components of *Dan Shen* are tanshinone, cryptotanshinone, miltirone, ß-sitosterol, and vitamin E.

Use of *Dan Shen* can help delay senility, enhance the immunologic function, dilate coronary arteries, strengthen the heart, lower blood pressure, regulate the function of blood platelets, resist tumors, combat bacteria, and tranquilize the mind. *Dan Shen* is prescribed as a tonic for building up health, retarding senility, and prolonging life.

Dan Shen is decocted in water for oral dose or taken in other dosage forms. The usual dosage is 5–15 grams.

San Qi (Radix notoginseng). *San Qi* is sweet and slightly bitter in taste and warm in nature. *San Qi* has the power to arrest bleeding, promote blood flow, remove blood stasis, relieve pain, and strengthen the body. It is used as a traditional blood-arresting drug to treat various kinds of hemorrhages such as traumatic injury and pain due to blood stasis and swelling.

Recently, it has been used effectively in the treatment of anemia, coronary heart disease, hyperlipernia, and hyperkinetic syndrome.

Modern research has found that *San Qi* contains the following main active elements similar to those of *Ren Shen (Radix Ginseng)*, which includes saponin, flavenoids, alkaloids, proteins, sugar, fatty oils, volatile oils, resin, nucleosides, and carotene.

Its pharmacological actions include nourishing the blood, improving the function of the cardiovascular system, regulating the immunologic function, adjusting (up or down) the blood sugar, arresting bleeding, resisting inflammation, tranquilizing the mind, and relieving pain. In short, *San Qi* is a good tonic for nourishment and healthcare.

Dried or prepared *San Qi* is ground into powder and is taken with boiled water. The dosage for dried *San Qi* is 1.0–1.5 grams of the powder or for the prepared, 3–5 grams. Alternatively, it may be soaked in liquor or infused in boiling water and taken as tea. The usual dosage is 3–10 grams.

Rhizoma gastrodiae. *Tian Ma* is sweet and mild-natured. It is used to calm internal wind, relieve convulsions, subdue exuberant *yang* of the liver, and tranquilize the mind. It has been traditionally used as a liver-wind-calming drug to treat dizziness, numbness of the limbs, and hemiplegia.

The main active elements of *Tian Ma* are gastrodine, vanillyl alcohol, succinic acid, ß-sitosterol, vitamin A-like substance, glucose, and alkaloids.

Pharmacological studies have indicated that *Tian Ma* has the power to enhance longevity. It is used to tranquilize the mind, alleviate pain, and relieve convulsions. It can enhance the immunologic function of the body, improve the nutritive blood flow in the cardiac muscles, and increase the hypoxiatolerance of experimental animals.

Tian Ma is decocted in water for oral use or ground into powder and swallowed in amounts of 1.0–1.5 grams with boiled water. Alternatively, it may be soaked in liquor or put into other dosage forms. The usual dosage of *Tian Ma* is 3–10 grams.

Hua Fen (Pollen). The reproductive cells in the stamens of flowers are collected and pollinated to the pistils by bees. The reproductive cells of the pistils are inseminated and a kind of pollen of nectar source is developed. *Hua Fen* is this pollen. *Hua Fen* is an ideal tonic for people who are old and healthy. It is used to prevent diseases, build up health, postpone senility, and promise longevity. *Hua Fen* is especially good for athletes, for improving a woman's looks, and for the treatment of neurosism, anemia, prostatic hyperplasia, diabetes, angiocardiopathy, ulcerous disorders, and menopausal syndrome.

Research has proved that *Hua Fen* contains 20 kinds of amino acids, 14 kinds of vitamins, 24 kinds of inorganic elements, 18 kinds of natural organized enzymes, fat, hormones, and aromatic substances.

The pharmacological actions of *Hua Fen* include activizing the hematopoietic functions, regulating cardiovascular functions, combating bacteria, resisting tumors, and delaying senility.

Hua Fen is often found in the form of a prepared product, and should be taken according to the accompanying instructions.

2.2 Commonly Used Chinese Patent Medicines for Healthcare

2.2.1 Patent Medicines for Tonifying *Qi*

BU ZHONG YI QI WAN

Main Ingredients
Huang Qi (Radix astragali)
Dang Shen (Radix codonopsis)
Gan Cao (Radix glycyrrhizae)
Dang Gui (Radix angelicae sinensis)
Chen Pi (Pericarpium citri reticulatae)
Sheng Ma (Rhizoma cimicifugae)

Chai Hu (Radix bupleuri)
Bai Zhu (Rhizoma atractylodis macrocephalae)
Dosage Form
Honeyed bolus or water-paste pill.
Dosage and Administration
Taken orally, twice daily, 9 grams each time.
Effect
Reinforces the middle *jiao*, replenishes *qi*, elevates the clear *qi* and sends down turbid indications.
Effects also include: headache and languor due to the hypofunction of both the spleen and the lungs, spontaneous sweating due to *yin* deficiency, aversion to wind, anorexia, chills or fever, dysentery, gastroptosis, metroptosis, syndromes of asthenia, various kinds of anemia, and gastritis.
Source
The book *Pi Wei Lun*

SHEN LING BAI ZHU WAN

Main Ingredients
Ren Shen (Radix ginseng)
Fu Ling (poria)
Bai Zhu (Rhizoma atractylodis macrocephalae)
Bai Bian Dou (Semen dolichoris album)
Shan Yao (Rhizoma dioscoreae)
Gan Cao (Radix glycyrrhizae)
Lian Zi (Semen nelumbinis)
Jie Geng (Radix platycodi)
Sha Ren (Fructus amomi)
Yi Yi Ren (Semen coicis)
Dosage Form
Water-paste pill.
Dosage and Administration
Taken orally, once or twice daily, 6–9 grams each time.
Effect
Nourishes the spleen and stomach and adjusts their functions.
Indications
Dyspepsia due to weakness of the spleen and stomach and manifested as vomiting or diarrhea, sallowness and emaciation, lassitude and hypodynamia, chronic nephritis.
Source
The book *Tai Ping Hui Min He Ji Ju Fang*

SI JUN ZI WAN

Main Ingredients
Dang Shen (Radix codonopsis)
Bai Zhu (Rhizoma atractylodis macrocephalae)
Fu Ling (poria)
Gan Cao (Radix glycyrrhizae)

Dosage Form
Water-paste pill.
Dosage and Administration
Taken 3 times daily, 6 grams each time.
Effect
Invigorates the spleen and replenishes *qi*.
Indications
Weakness of the spleen and stomach, manifested as poor appetite, loose stools, sallow complexion, dizziness and debility including chronic gastroenteritis, gastric and duodenal ulcers, protracted or chronic hepatitis, anemia, and leukocytopenia.
Source
The book *Tai Ping Hui Min He Ji Ju Fang*

SHI QUAN DA BU WAN

Ingredients
Dang Shen (Radix codonopsis)
Huang Qi (Radix astragali)
Rou Gui (cortex cinnamorni)
Shu Di (Rhizoma rehmanniae praeparata)
Bai Zhu (Rhizoma atractylodis macrocephalae)
Dang Gui (Radix angelicae sinensis)
Bai Shao (Radix paeoniae alba)
Chuan Xiong (Rhizoma chuanxiong)
Fu Ling (Poria)
Gan Cao (Radix glycyrrhizae)
Dosage Form
Honeyed bolus, 1 bolus weighs 9 grams
Dosage and Administration
Taken orally, twice daily, 1 bolus each time.
Effect
Invigorates the spleen and replenishes *qi*, enriches the blood, and regulates the nutrient system.
Indications
Syndrome due to deficiency of both *qi* and blood, marked by general debility, sallow complexion, asthma and cough due to consumption, lassitude, spermatorrhea, impairment of blood, and weakness of the loins and knees.
Source
The book *Tai Ping Hui Min He Ji Ju Fang*

LIANG SHEN JING

Main Ingredients
Ren Shen (Radix ginseng)
Wu Jia Shen (Radlix acanthopanacis senticosil)
Dosage Form
Oral liquid, each ampule contains 10 mls of liquid.

Dosage and Administration

Taken orally before breakfast, 1 ampule each day.

Effect

Replenishes *qi*, enriches the blood, and strengthens the constitution.

Indications

Neurosism, infirmity with age, general debility after illness, anorexia, heart failure, hepatitis, and anemia.

Manufacturer

Yanji No. 2 Pharmaceutical Factory

Notes

Regular intake can help the body resist disease.

REN SHEN FENG WANG JIANG (SHUANG BAO SU KOU FU YE)

Main Ingredients

Ren Shen (Radix ginseng)
Feng Wang Jiang (Royal Jelly)
Feng Mi (Mel)

Dosage Form

Honey jelly, each ampule containing 10 mls.

Dosage and Administration

Taken orally, twice daily, 1 ampule each time.

Effect

Builds up the body, replenishes *qi*, strengthens the spleen.

Indications

Weak constitution, debility after illness, malnutrition, neurosism, lassitude, poor appetite, and decline of neurometabolism.

Manufacturer

Bei Jing Dong Feng Pharmaceutical Factory and Hangzhou No. 2 Pharmaceutical Factory of Traditional Chinese Medicines.

Notes

Regular intake will promote growth and development, improve physical and mental ability, prevent disease, and prolong life. *Shuang Bao Su Kou Fu Ye* is manufactured by Hangzhou No. 2 factory of Traditional Chinese Medicines. Its ingredients and effects are basically the same as those of *Ren Shen Feng Wang Jiang*.

BEI JING FENG WANG JING

Ingredients

Feng Wang Jiang (Royal Jelly)
Ren Shen (Radix ginseng)
Dang Shen (Radix codonopsis)
Gou Qi Zi (Fructus lycii)
Wu Wei Zi (Fructus schisandrae)

Dosage Form

Oral liquid, each ampule, contains 10 mls of liquid.

Dosage and Administration

Take orally in the morning or before going to bed in the evening, 1 ampule daily.

Effect

Invigorates the spleen, replenishes *qi*, and promotes the production of body fluids.

Indications

Anorexia, neurosis, anemia, gastric ulcers, senility, hepatitis, arthritis, angiitis.

Manufacturer

Beijing Nutrient Medicine Factory

Notes

This medicine is a tonic of high quality.

YAN NIAN YI SHOU JING

Ingredients

The same as those in the prescription of *Yan Nian Yi Shou Dan*, a secret recipe from the Institute of Imperial Physicians in the Qing dynasty.

Dosage Form

Oral liquid, each ampule containing 10 mls of liquid.

Dosage and Administration

Take orally in the morning or before going to bed in the evening, 1–2 times daily, 1 ampule each time.

Effect

Regulates the metabolism of the body and slows down histiocytic decay and senility of the old.

Indications

Senility and general debility.

Manufacturer

Wuhan Zhonglian Pharmaceutical Factory

Notes

Produced according to traditional extractive process.

WU JIA SHEN CHONG JI

Main Ingredients

Wu Jia Shen (Radix acanthopanacis senticosi)

Dosage Form

Granules in lumps for infusing, each lump weighs 12.25 grams.

Dosage and Administration

Taken orally after being infused with boiling water, twice daily, 1 lump each time.

Effect

Strengthens the body's resistance and restores the normal function of the body to consolidate the constitution, tranquilize the mind, and improve mental power.

Indications

Neurosism, debility after illness, lassitude, insomnia, anorexia, coronary heart disease, and leukopenia.

Manufacturer

Haerbin No. 1 Pharmaceutical Factory of Traditional Chinese Medicines

DA LI SHI BU YE

Main Ingredients

Wu Jia Shen (Radix acanthopanacis senticosi)

Huang Qi (Radix astragah)

Dan Shen (Radix salviae miltiorrhizae)

Dosage Form

Syrup in 500 ml. bottle.

Dosage and Administration

Taken orally, 3 times daily, 20 ml. each time.

Effect

Strengthens the body, improves mental power, tranquilizes the mind.

Indications

Weak constitution, debility after illness, lassitude, soreness and weakness of the loins and knees, dizziness, severe palpitations, and insomnia.

Manufacturer

Experimental Pharmaceutical Factory of Heilongjiang Institute of Traditional Chinese Medicine

REN SHEN ZI BU PIAN VITAMIN C

Main Ingredients

Ren Shen (Radix ginseng)

Vitamin C

Dosage Form

Tablet form

Dosage and Administration

Taken orally, 3 times daily, 3–5 tablets each time.

Effect

Invigorates *qi* to build up health.

Indications

Infirmity with age, disorders in the convalescence, dyspnea due to deficiency of the lungs, diarrhea due to deficiency of the spleen, neurosism, amnesia, anorexia, chronic hepatitis, diabetes, anemia, hypertension,and syndrome due to deficiency of Vitamin C.

Manufacturer

Beijing Pharmaceutical Factory

Main Ingredients
Ren Shen (Radix ginseng)
Tian Dong (Radix asparagi)
Shu Di Huang (Rhizoma rehmanniae praeparata)

Effect
Invigorates *qi*, nourishes *yin*, replenishes the vital essence and blood.

Indications
Deficiency of vital essence, *qi* and blood in the middle aged and the elderly, general debility, and weakness in the convalescence.

Manufacturer
Hangzhou No. 2 Pharmaceutical Factory of Traditional Chinese Medicine

Main Ingredients
Ren Shen (Radix ginseng)
Tai Zi Shen (Radix pseudostellariae)
Dang Shen (Radix codonopsis)
Feng Wang Jiang (Royal Jelly)
Mai Dong (Radix ophiopogonis)
Zhi Shou Wu (Radix polygoni multiflori preparata)
Dang Gui (Radix angelicae sinensis)

Dosage Form
Oral liquid, 1 ampule containing 10 mls.

Dosage and Administration
Taken orally, once daily, 1 ampule each time.

Effect
Invigorates the spleen, replenishes *qi*, nourishes *yin*, enriches blood.

Indications
Deficiency of both *qi* and blood, *yin*-deficiency of the liver and kidney, insufficiency of body fluid, weakness in the convalescence, and infirmity with age.

Manufacturer
Wuxi Pharmaceutical Factory of Traditional Chinese Medicine

2.2.2 PATENT MEDICINES FOR NOURISHING BLOOD

Source
The book *Rui Zhu Tang Jing Yan Fang*

Ingredients
Ren Shen (Radix ginseng)
Shu Di Huang (Rhizoma rehmanniae praeparata)

Dang Gui (Radix angelicae sinensis)
Bai Shao (Radix paeoiae alba)
Chuan Xiong (rhizoma chuanxiong)
Fu Ling (Poria)
Bai Zhu (Rhizoma atractylodis macrocephalae)
Gan Cao (Radix glycyrrhizae)

Dosage Form
Bolus, each bolus weighs 9 grams.

Dosage and Administration
Taken orally, twice daily, 2 boluses each time.

Effect
Regulates and invigorates *qi* and blood.

Indications
Pallid countenance and thin shape, anorexia, weakness of the limbs, dizziness, blurring of vision due to deficiency of *qi* and blood, irregular menstruation, various kinds of anemia, primary thrombocytopenic purpura, and rheumatic heart disease.

FU FANG E JIAO JIANG

Main Ingredients
E Jiao (Colla corii asini)
Ren Shen (Radix ginseng)
Shan Zha (Fructus crataegi)

Dosage Form
Honey jelly

Dosage and Administration
Taken orally, 3 times daily, 20 ml. each time.

Effect
Replenishes *qi*, nourishes blood.

Indications
Syndrome due to deficiency of *qi* and blood, anemia, and leukopenia.
Intake may help nourish health and prolong life.

Manufacturer
Shandong Donge Ejiao Factory

KANG BAO

Main Ingredients
Ci Wu Jia (Radix acanthopanacis senticosi)
Feng Wang Jiang (Royal Jelly)
Yin Yang Huo (Herba epimedii)
Gou Qi (Fructus lycii)
Huang Jing (Radix polygonati)
Shu Di (Rhizoma rehmanniae praeparata)
Huang Qi (Radix astragali)
Shan Zha (Fructus crataegi)

Dosage Form
Honey jelly, each bottle containing 100 mls.
Dosage and Administration
Taken orally, 5–10 ml. each time.
Effect
Invigorates *qi*, enriches the blood, warms the kidneys, replenishes the vital essence, resists senility.
Indications
Syndrome due to deficiency of both *qi* and blood, anemia, and infirmity with age.
It may be used by the healthy to prevent disease and preserve health.
Manufacturer
Shandong Yantai Pharmaceutical Factory of Traditional Chinese Medicines

SHEN QI WANG JIANG YANG XUE JING

Main Ingredients
Feng Wang Jiang (Royal Jelly)
Ren Shen Jing (extracts of the ingredient *Radix ginseng*)
Huang Qi Jing (extracts of the ingredient *Radix astragali*)
Dosage Form
Oral liquid, each ampule contains 10 mls.
Dosage and Administration
Taken orally before breakfast, once daily, 1 ampule each time.
Effect
Enriches the blood, replenishes *qi*, strengthens the heart, and invigorates the spleen.
Indications
Anemia, general debility, infirmity with age, neurosism, hepatitis, and baldness.
Manufacturer
Yanji No. 2 Pharmaceutical Factory in Jilin Province

REN SHEN SHOU WU JING

Main Ingredients
Hong Shen (Radix ginseng rubra)
He Shou Wu (Radix polygoni-multiflori)
Dosage Form
Oral liquid, each ampule contains 50 mls.
Dosage and Administration
Taken orally, 3 times daily, 10 ml. each time.
Effect
Enriches the blood, replenishes *qi*, tranquilizes the mind, improves mental power.
Indications
Deficiency of both *qi* and blood, amnesia, insomnia, anorexia, lassitude, impotence, and prospermia.

Main Ingredients
E Jiao (Colla corii asini)
Dang Shen (Radix codonopsis)
Shu Di (Rhizoma rehmanniae praeparata)

Dosage Form
Granules for infusing

Dosage and Administration
Taken orally after being infused with boiling water, twice daily, 20 grams each time.

Effect
Nourishes the liver and kidneys, invigorates *qi* and blood.

Indications
Deficiency of both *qi* and blood, weakness of the body, and infirmity.

Main Ingredients
Dang Shen (Radix codonopsis)
Shu Di (Rhizoma rehmanniae praeparata)

Dosage Form
Granules for infusing, each tube contains 250 grams.

Dosage and Administration
Taken orally after being infused with boiling water, twice daily 20 grams each time.

Effect
Replenishes *qi*, nourishes blood.

Indications
Deficiency of both *Qi* and blood, general debility, and weakness in convalescence.

Main Ingredients
Ren Shen (Radix ginseng)
He Shou Wu (Radix polygoni multiflori)
Quan Dang Gui (Radix angelicae sinensis)
Bai Fu Ling (Poria)
Jin ying Zi (Fructus rosae laevigatae)

Dosage Form
Syrup, each bottle contains 300 ml.

Dosage and Administration
Taken orally, twice daily, 20 ml. each time.

Effect
Replenishes *qi*, nourishes blood, strengthens the spleen, and tonifies the kidney.

Indications

Deficiency of *qi* and blood, general debility, and early graying of hair.

Regular intake will enrich the blood, nourish the heart, strengthen the tendons and bones, darken the hair and regulate menstruation.

BU XUE NING SHEN PIAN

Main Ingredients

Shou Wu Teng (Caulis polygoni multiflori)
Ji Xue Teng (Caulis spatholobi)
Shu Di (Rhizoma rehmanniae praeparata)

Dosage Form

Tablets

Dosage and Administration

Taken orally, 3 times daily, 5 tablets each time.

Effect

Enriches the blood, tranquilizes the mind, nourishes *yin*, and tonifies the kidneys.

Indications

Insomnia, amnesia, nocturnal emission, frequent urination, soreness and weakness of the loins and knees, and irregular menstruation.

Manufacturer

Guangzhou Hongwei Pharmaceutical Factory

SHEN GUI ZAO ZHI

Main Ingredients

Hong Zao (Fructus jujubae)
Tai Zi Shen (Radix pseudostellariae)
Dang Gui (Radix angelicae sinensis)

Dosage Form

Honey syrup

Dosage and Administration

Taken orally with warm boiled water, 2–3 times daily, 10–20 ml. each time.

Effect

Nourishes the blood, promotes the production of body fluids, replenishes *qi*, and strengthens the spleen.

Indications

Deficiency of both *qi* and blood, listlessness, general debility, poor appetite, and various consumptive disorders.

Manufacturer

Benbu Pharmaceutical Factory of Traditional Chinese Medicines in Anhui Province

2.2.3 Patent Medicines for Supporting Yang

Source

The book *Jin Kui Yao Lüe*

Main Ingredients

Shu Di (Rhizoma rehmanniae praeparata)
Shan Yao (Radix dioscoreae)
Rou Gui (Cortex cinnamomi)
Dan Pi (Cortex moutan)
Fu Ling (Poria)
Fu Zi (Radix Aconiti lateralis preparata)
Shan Yu Rou (Fructus cornii)
Ze Xie (Rhizoma alismatis)

Dosage Form

Honeyed bolus, each bolus weighs 9 grams.

Dosage and Administration

Taken orally, twice daily, 1 bolus each time.

Effect

Warms the kidney-*yang*.

Indications

Syndrome due to deficiency of the kidney-*yang*, deficiency type of the spleen and stomach marked by soreness and weakness of the loins and legs, spasmodic sensation of the lower abdomen, seminal emission, loose stools, frequent urination, and edema of the lower limbs.

Main Ingredients

Hai Long (Syngnathus)
Ge Jie (Gecko)
Bei Qi (Radix astragali)
Ren Shen (Radix ginseng)
Shou Wu (Radix polygoni multiflori)
Dang Gui (Radix angelicae sinensis)
Qi Zi (Fructus lycii)
Chen Xiang (Lignum aquilariae resinatum)

Dosage Form

Oral liquid, each ampule contains 10 mls.

Dosage and Administration

Taken orally, 1–2 times daily, 1 ampule each time.

Effect

Tonifies the body, replenishes *qi*, enriches the blood, strengthens the heart, brightens the face, improves eyesight.

Indications

Neurosism, overstrain, deficiency of *qi* and blood, soreness of the loins, pain in the back, weakness of the limbs, dizziness, and blurred vision.

Notes

This medicine is a high quality tonic. It is especially useful for the elderly.

Manufacturer

Jinan Pharmaceutical Factory of Traditional Chinese Medicines in Shandong Province, China

NAN BAO

Main Ingredients

Lü Shen (Peniet testes asini)
Gou Shen (Peniet testes canini)
Hai Ma (Hippocampus)
Ren Shen (Radix ginseng)
Lu Rong (Cornu cervi pantotrichum)
E Jiao (Colla corii asini)
Huang Qi (Radix astragali)
Shan Yu Rou (Fructus corni)

Dosage Form

Capsules, each weighs 0.3 grams.

Dosage and Administration

Taken orally, twice daily, 2–3 capsules each time.

Effect

Warms the kidney-*yang*, replenishes *qi*, and builds up the body.

Indications

Syndrome due to deficiency of the kidney-*Yang*, marked by impotence, spermatorrhea, weakness and soreness of the loins and knees, cold and damp feeling of scrotum, listlessness, and anorexia.

Manufacturer

Houma Pharmaceutical Factory of Traditional Chinese Medicines in Shanxi Province

SHEN RONG BIAN WAN

Main Ingredients

Ren Shen (Radix ginseng)
Lu Rong (Cornu cervi pantotrichum)
Diao Bian (Peniet testes martes)
Hai Ma (Hippocampus)
Du Zhong (Cortex eucommiae)
Gou Qi (Fructus lycii)
Rou Gui (Cortex cinnamomi)

Dosage Form

Water-paste pill

Dosage and Administration

Taken according to the instructions

Effect

Tonifies the kidneys, supports *yang*, strengthens vital essence, and promotes the production of marrow.

Indications
Weakened *qi* due to deficiency of the kidney, impotence, prospermia emission, and all disorders due to deficiency of the kidney in men or women.

Manufacturer
Dalian Pharmaceutical Factory of Traditional Chinese Medicines

YANG CHUN YAO

Main Ingredients
Shui Diao Bian (Peniet testes martes)
Mei Lu Bian (Peniet testes cervi)
Guang Gou Bian (Peniet testes canini)
Lu Rong (Cornu cervi pantotrichum)
Yin Yang Huo (Herba epimedii)
Ba Ji Tian (Radix morindae officinalis)
Huang Qi (Radix astragali)
Fei Yang Qi Shi (Actinolitum refined with water)
Tu Si Zi (Semen cuscutae)
He Shou Wu (Radix polygoni multiflori)
Rou Cong Rong (Herba cistanchis)
Shan Yao (Rhizoma dioscoreae)

Dosage Form
Capsules

Dosage and Administration
Taken orally, twice daily, 2 capsules each time.

Effect
Strengthens the loins, supports *yang*, restores *qi*, and builds up health.

Indications
Weak constitution, emission due to physical debility, lassitude, dizziness, tinnitus, palpitations caused by fright, amnesia, soreness and weakness of the loins and knees, decline of memory, neurosis, insomnia, and anorexia.

YI SHEN TANG JIANG

Main Ingredients
Gou Qi Zi (Fructus lycii)
Fu Pen Zi (Fructus riibi)
Wu Wei Zi (Fructus schisandrae)

Dosage Form
Syrup

Dosage and Administration
Taken orally, twice daily, 5–10 ml. each time.

Effect
Reinforces kidney-*yang*, replenishes the vital essence, and supplements marrow.

Indications
General debility, impotence due to deficiency of the kidney, nocturnal emissions, and turbid urine.
Manufacturer
Tianjin No. I Pharmaceutical Factory of Traditional Chinese Medicines

SHEN RONG DA BU WAN

Main Ingredients
Sheng Shai Shen (dried Radix ginseng)
Lu Rong (Cornu cervi pantotrichum)
Rou Cong Rong (Herba cistanchis)
Lu. Jiao Jiao (Colla cornus cervi)
Suo Yang (Herba cynomorii)
Chen Xiang (Lignum aquilariae resinatum)
Rou Gui (Cortex cinnamomi)
Fu Zi (Radix Aconiti lateralis preparata)
Tu Si Zi (Semen cuscutae)
Gou Qi Zi (Fructus lycii)
Du Zhong (Cortex eucommiae)
Shou Wu (Radix polygoni multiflori)
Shan Yao (Rhizoma dioscoreae)
Fu Ling (Poria)
Yuan Zhi (Radix polygalae)
Dosage Form
Honeyed bolus, each bolus weighs 3.2 grams.
Dosage and Administration
Taken orally, 1–2 times daily, 1 bolus each time.
Effect
Tonifies kidney-*yang*, promotes the production of vital essence, and replenishes marrow.
Indications
Cold syndrome of the stomach due to *yang*-deficiency, soreness and weakness of the loins and knees, impotence, emission, prosperinia, spermatorrhea, and frequent urination.
Notes
It is prepared according to the prescription from Zhejiang.

CHU FENG JING

Main Ingredients
Ji Tai (chicken embryo)
Yang Bian (Peniet testes caprae seu ovis)
Ren Shen (Radix ginseng)
Sha Ren (Fructus amomi)
Huang Qi (Radix astragali)
Gou Qi (Fructus lycii)
Yin Yang Huo (Herba epimedii)

Lu Rong (Cornu cervi pantotrichum)
Rou Gui (Cortex cinnamomi)
Dang Gui (Radix angelicae sinensis)
Rou Cong Rong (Herba cistanchis)

Dosage Form
Oral liquid, each ampule contains 10 mls.

Dosage and Administration
Taken orally, twice daily, 1 ampule each time.

Effect
Tonifies the kidney-*yang*, strengthens the loins, builds up health, replenishes *qi*, and enriches the blood.

Indications
Syndrome due to deficiency of the kidney-*yang*, anemia, soreness of the loins, pain in the back, weakness of the limbs, dizziness, tinnitus, neurosism, insomnia, palpitations, overtaxation of the mind, decline of memory, poor appetite, reduced sexual function or coldness in the womb, and irregular menstruation.

Manufacturer
Jinan Pharmaceutical Factory of Traditional Chinese Medicines in Shandong Province of China

Notes
This medicine is a high quality strong tonic.

HAI MA BU SHEN WAN

Main Ingredients
Hai Ma (Hippocampus)
Ren Shen (Radix ginseng)
Hua Long Gu (Os draconis)
Gou Qi Zi (Fructus lycii)
Hei Lü Shen (Peniet testes asini)
Lu Jin (Ligamentum cervi)
Bu Gu Zhi (Fructus psoraleae)
Fu Ling (Poria)
Huang Qi (Radix astragali)
He Tao Ren (Semen juglandis)
Lu Rong (Cornu cervi pantotrichum)
Ge Jie Wei (tails of gecko)
Hai Gou Shen (Peniet testes callorhini)
Xian Dui Xia (fresh prawns)
Hu Gu (Os tigris)
Hua Lu Shen (Peniet testes cervi)
Shan Yu Rou (Fructus corni)
Dang Gui (Radix angelicae sinensis)

Dosage Form
Pills. 10 pills weigh 2.7 grams.

Dosage and Administration
Taken orally on an empty stomach, twice daily, 10 pills each time.

Effect

Supplements kidney-*yang*, reinforces the brain, and strengthens the body.

Indications

Syndrome due to deficiency of both *qi* and blood as well as insufficiency of kidney-*qi*, marked by general debility, sallow complexion, emaciation, palpitation, short breath, weakness of the loins and legs, and impotence.

Manufacturer

Tianjin No. 3 Pharmaceutical Factory of Traditional Chinese Medicines

MEI HUA LU RONG XUE

Main Ingredients

Lu Rong Xue (Sanguis cervi)
Mei Hua Lu Rong (Cornu cervi pantotrichum)
Wu Jia Shen (Radix acanthopanacis senticosi)

Dosage Form

Oral liquid, each ampule contains 10 mls.

Dosage and Administration

Taken orally before breakfast, once daily, 1 ampule each time.

Effect

Warms kidney-*yang*, promotes the production of vital essence, and enriches the blood.

Indications

Male hypogonadism, irregular menstruation, coldness in the womb, leucorrhagia with reddish and whitish discharge, copos, postpartum debility, infirmity with age, weakness of the heart, malnutrition, anemia, overtaxation of the mind, hyponinesis, soreness and weakness of the loins and knees, dizziness, and insomnia.

HAI SHEN WAN

Main Ingredients

Hai Shen (Holothuriae)
Hu Tao Rou (Semen juglandis)
Yang Yao Zi (Peniet testes caprae seu ovis)
Zhu Ji Sui (spinal cord of pig)
Lu Bao Jiao (Colla comus cervi)
Gui Ban (Carapax plastruin testudinis)
Du Zhong (Cortex eucommiae)
Niu Xi (Radix achyranthis bidentatae)
Ba Ji Tian (Radix morindae officinalis)
Tu Si Zi (Semen cuscutae)
Bu Gu Zhi (Fructus psoraleae)
Gou Qi Zi (Fructus lycii)
Dang Gui (Radix angelicae sinensis)

Dosage Form
Honeyed bolus, each bolus weighs 9 grams.
Dosage and Administration
Taken orally, twice daily, 1 bolus each time.
Effect
Reinforces kidney-*yang*, nourishes the blood, and replenishes the vital essence.
Indications
Syndrome due to deficiency of the kidney-*yang* manifested as impotence, emission, soreness and weakness of the loins and knees, dizziness, tinnitus, and weakness of the limbs.

2.2.4 PATENT MEDICINES FOR NOURISHING *YIN*

LIU WEI DI HUANG WAN

Source
The book *Xiao Er Yao Zheng Zhi Jue*
Ingredients
Shu Di Huang (Rhizoma rehmanniae praeparata)
Shan Yao (Rhizoma dioscoreae)
Shan Yu Rou (Fructus corni)
Fu Ling (poria)
Ze Xie (Rhizoma alismatis)
Dan Pi (Cortex moutan)
Dosage Form
Honeyed boluses, 1 bolus weighs 9 grams.
Dosage and Administration
Taken orally, twice daily, 1 bolus each time.
Effect
Tonifies the liver and kidneys.
Indications
Syndrome due to *yin*-deficiency of the liver and kidneys marked by soreness and weakness of the loins and legs, dizziness, tinnitus, insomnia, nocturnal emission, dry mouth in diabetes, hectic fever, night sweating, and dysphoria with feverish sensations in the chest, palms, and soles.

REN SHEN GU BEN WAN

Ingredients
Ren Shen (Radix ginseng)
Shan Yao (Rhizoma dioscoreae)
Shu Di Huang (Rhizoma rehmanniae praeparata)
Tian Dong (Radix asparagi)
Mai Dong (Radix ophiopogonis)
Shan Zhu Yu (Fructus corni)
Feng Mi (Mel)
Fu Ling (Poria)
Dosage Form
Honeyed bolus, 1 bolus weighs 9 grams.

Dosage and Administration
Taken orally, twice daily, 1 bolus each time.
Effect
Nourishes *yin*, supplements the blood, replenishes *qi*, and promotes the production of body fluids.
Indications
Syndrome due to *yin*-deficiency and weakened *qi* marked by general debility, palpitations, shortness of breath, pain in the loins, tinnitus, soreness and weakness of the limbs, and hectic fever due to consumption.

JIAN NAO CHONG JI

Main Ingredients
Gou Qi Zi (Fructus lycii)
Suan Zao Ren (Semen ziziphi spinosae)
Dosage Form
Granules for infusing, each bag contains 14 grams.
Dosage and Administration
Take orally before going to bed in the evening, once daily, 1 bag each time.
Effect
Replenishes the kidney-*yin*, strengthens the brain, nourishes the heart, and calms the mind.
Indications
Yin-deficiency of the liver and the kidney, neurosism, insomnia, amnesia, dizziness, tinnitus, and soreness and weakness of the loins.

SHEN QI FENG HUANG JIANG

Main Ingredients
Feng Ru (Lac regis apis)
Feng Mi (Mel)
Dang Shen (Radix codonopsis)
Gou Qi Zi (Fructus lycii)
Dosage Form
Honey jelly, each ampule contains 10 mls.
Dosage and Administration
Taken orally, 1–2 times daily, 1 ampule each time.
Effect
Tonifies the liver and kidneys, replenishes *qi*, and improves acuity of vision.
Indications
Yin-deficiency of the liver and kidney, dizziness, blurring of vision, soreness and weakness of the loins and knees, poor appetite, lassitude, infirmity with age, and debility in convalescence.

ZI YIN BAI BU WAN

Main Ingredients
Dang Gui (Radix angelicae sinensis)
Fu Ling (Poria)
Yuan Zhi (Radix polygalae)
Niu Xi (Radix achyranthis bidentatae)
Mai Dong (Radix ophiopogonis)
Zhi Mu (Rhizoma anemarrhenae)
Rou Cong Rong (Herba cistanchis)
Gou Qi Zi (Fructus lycii)
Nü Zhen Zi (Fructus ligustri lucidi)
Tu Si Zi (Semen cuscutae)
Suo Yang (Herba cynomorii)
Ba Ji Tian (Radix morindea officinalis)
Bai Zi Ren (Seffien biotae)
Shan Yu Rou (Fructus corni)

Dosage Form
Honeyed bolus, each weighing 3–9 grams.

Dosage and Administration
Taken orally, twice daily, 6–9 grams each time.

Effect
Tonifies the kidneys, replenishes *yin*, controls nocturnal emissions, and calms the mind.

Indications
Interior heat due to *yin*-deficiency, dizziness, lassitude, soreness in the loins, weakness of the limbs, night sweats, and infirmity with age.

KANG FU WAN

Main Ingredients
Tai Zi Shen (Radix beudostellariae)
Dang Gui (Radix angelicae sinensis)
Wu Wei Zi (Fructus schisandrae)
Zhen Zhu Mu (Concha margaritifera usta)
Shan Yao (Rhizoma dioscoreae)
Shu Di (Rhizma rehmanniae praeparata)
Chuan Duan (Radix disaci)

Dosage Form
Water-pills

Dosage and Administration
Taken orally, 3 times daily, 10 pills each time.

Effect
Tonifies the kidneys, restores *qi*, nourishes the blood to control nocturnal emissions, and builds up health.

Indications
General debility, in the convalescence, *yin*-deficiency of the liver and kidney, dizziness, tinnitus, lassitude in the loins, insomnia, amnesia, emission, and night sweats.

Manufacturer
Xian Pharmaceutical Factory of Traditional Chinese Medicines

QING GONG SHOU TAO WAN

Main Ingredients
Yi Zhi Ren (Fructus alpiniae oxyphyllae)
Da Sheng Di (Radix rehmanniae)
Gou Qi Zi (Fructus lycii)
Tian Dong (Radix asparagi)
Ren Shen (Radix ginseng)
Dang Gui (Radix aftelicae sinensis)
He Tao Rou (Semen juglandis)

Dosage Form
Honeyed boluses, each weighing 6 grams.

Dosage and Administration
Taken orally, twice daily, 1 bolus each time.

Effect
Reinforces the kidneys, invigorates primordial *qi*, nourishes *yin*, supports *yang*, enriches blood, and prolongs life.

Indications
Infirmity with age, debility in the convalescence, various and disorders of deficiency type.

Manufacturer
Darentang Pharmaceutical Factory in Tianjin City

Notes
This medicine is produced according to a secret prescription from the Palace of the Qing dynasty. It is a good tonic for resisting senility and enhancing longevity.

2.2.5 OTHER PATENT MEDICINES FOR HEALTHCARE

LING ZHI PIAN

Main Ingredients
Ling Zhi (Ganoderma lucidum seu japonicum)

Dosage Form
Tablets or granules to be used for infusion. Each tablet weighs 1 grams; the granules are in lumps and each lump weighs 13 grams.

Dosage and Administration
The tablets are taken twice daily, 1–2 tablets each time. The granules are taken after being infused with boiling water, once daily, 1 lump each time.

Effect
Tonifies the heart, calms the mind, strengthens the spleen, regulates the stomach, builds up health, and prolongs life.

Indications
Neurosism, dizziness, insomnia, anorexia, coronary heart disease, and hyperlipemia.

Manufacturer
The Pharmaceutical Factory of Guangxi College of Traditional Chinese Medicine

YI NAO FU JIAN WAN

Main Ingredients
San Qi (Radix notoginseng)
Xi Hong Hua (Stigma croci)
Chuan Xiong (Rhizoma chuanxiong)

Dosage Form
Capsules, each capsule weighs 0.3 grams.

Dosage and Administration
Taken orally, 3 times daily, 6–8 capsules each time.

Effect
Supplements the brain to benefit the mind, smooths the channels and collaterals, activates the blood circulation to remove stasis, and eliminates phlegm to induce resuscitation.

Indications
Distortion of the face, herniparalysis, and dysphasia due to acute ischeinic apoplexy.

NAO LING SU

Main Ingredients
Ren Shen (Radix ginseng)
Lu Rong (Cornu cervi pantotrichum)
Gui Ban (Carapax plastrum testudinis)
Lu Jiao Jiao (Colla cornus cervi)
Suan Zao Ren (Semen ziziphi spinosae)
Gou Qi Zi (Fructus lycii)
Wu Wei Zi (Fructus schisandrae)
Fu Ling (Poria)
Yuan Zhi (Radix polygalae)

Dosage Form
Sugar coated tablets, each weighing 0.5 grams.

Dosage and Administration
Taken orally, twice daily, 2–3 tablets each time.

Effect
Supplements both *qi* and blood, nourishes the heart and kidneys, strengthens the brain, and calms the mind.

Indications
Neurosism, amnesia, insomnia, dizziness, blurring of vision, palpitation, shortness of breath, lassitude, general debility, spontaneous sweating, impotence, and seminal emissions.

Manufacturer
Jiamusi Pharmaceutical Factory of Traditional Chinese Medicines and Linyi Health Pharmaceutical Factory in Shandong Province.

Main Ingredients

Yin Er (Tremella)
Wu Jia Shen (Radix acanthopanacis senticosi)
Wu Wei Zi (Fructus schisandrae)
Dan Shen (Radix salviae miltiorrhizae)
Ban Lan Gen (Radix isatidis)
Gan Cao (Radix glycyrrhizae)

Dosage Form

Malt extract in lumps, each lump weighs 5.2 grams.

Dosage and Administration

Taken orally, 2–3 times daily, 1–2 lumps each time.

Effect

Restores the normal function of the body to consolidate the constitution, enriches the blood, tranquilizes the mind, clears away heat and toxic material, enhances the body's resistance, combats and prevents influenza and hepatitis, promotes growth and development, invigorates primordial *qi* and builds up the constitution in adults who take it regularly.

Manufacturer

Weihai Pharmaceutical Factory of Traditional Chinese Medicines in Shandong Province

Main Ingredients

Dan Shen (Radix salviae miltiorrhizae)
Wu Wei Zi (Fructus schisandrae)
Shi Chang Pu (Rgraminei)
He Huan Pi (Cortex albiziae)
Mo Han Lian (Herba ecliptae)
Nü Zhen Zi (Fructus ligustri lucidi)
Shou Wu Teng (Caulis polygoni multiflori)
Sheng Di (Radix rehmanniae)
Zhen Zhu Mu (Concha margaritifera usta)

Dosage Form

Pills

Dosage and Administration

Taken orally, 3 times daily, 15 pills each time.

Effect

Replenishes *yin*, nourishes the blood, tonifies the heart, and calms the mind.

Indications

Palpitations, insomnia, dizziness, and tinnitus.

Manufacturer

Shanghai No. 1 Pharmaceutical Factory of Traditional Chinese Medicines

Main Ingredients

Lu Rong (Cornu cervi pantotrichum)
Feng Wang Jiang (Royal Jelly)
Ci Wu Jia (Radix acanthopanacis senticosi)

Dosage Form

Oral liquid, each ampule contains 10 mls.

Dosage and Administration

Take orally after getting up in the morning or before going to bed in the evening, once daily, 1 ampule each time.

Effect

Reinforces the heart, strengthens the spleen, tonifies the kidneys, calms the mind, replenishes *qi*, and nourishes the blood.

Indications

Neurosism, deficiency of energy, poor appetite, dysplasia, infirmity with age, postpartum debility, and copos.

Notes

This medicine may be used for healthcare of athletes and children.

Main Ingredients

Ren Shen (Radix ginseng)
Ling Zhi (Ganoderma lucidum, seu japonicum)
Lu Rong (Cornu cervi pantotrichum)
Hong Hua (Flos carthami)
Dan Shen (Radix salviae miltiorrhizae)
Dan Pi (Cortex moutan)
Chuan Xiong (Rhizoma chuanxiong)
E Jiao (Colla corii asini)

Dosage Form

Capsules, each weighing 0.3 grams.

Dosage and Administration

Taken orally, 3 times daily, 4 capsules each time.

Effect

Replenishes *qi*, activates blood circulation, nourishes *yin*, supports *yang*, regulates menstruation, and treats leukorrhagia.

Indications

Irregular menstruation, dysmenorrhea, amenorrhea, leukorrhagia, sterility due to cold uterus, postpartum disorders, deficiency of vital essence due to consumption in males, and weakness of the loins and knees.

Manufacturer

Pharmaceutical Factory of Changchun College of Traditional Chinese Medicine and Dongfeng Pharmaceutical Factory in Jilin Province

Notes

It is a newly developed medicine for women's healthcare.

GENG NIAN AN

Main Ingredients

Shu Di (Rhizonia rehmanniae praeparata)
He Shou Wu (Radix polygoni multiflori)

Dosage and Administration

Taken according to the instructions

Effect

Replenishes *qi*, nourishes the blood, and strengthens health.

Indications

Neurosism, dizziness, tinnitus, restlessness, insomnia, poor appetite, anemia, sallow complexion, and general debility.

DAN QI PIAN

Main Ingredients

San Qi (Radix notoginseng)
Dan Shen (Radix salviae miltiorrhizae)

Dosage Form

Tablets

Dosage and Administration

Taken orally, 3 times daily, 3 tablets each time.

Effect

Reinforces the heart, dilates the coronary arteries, activates blood circulation, and removes stasis.

Indications

Neurosism and angina pectoris due to coronary heart disease.

Manufacturer

Tongrentang Pharmaceutical Factory in Beijing

NÜ BAO

Main Ingredients

Ren Shen (Radix ginseng)
Lu Tai (Fetus cervi)
Lu Rong (Cornu cervi pantotrichum)
Hong Hua (Flos carthami)
Dan Shen (Radix salviae miltiorrhizae)
Dan Pi (Cortex moutan)
Chuan Xiong (Rhizoma chuanxiong)
E Jiao (Colla corii asini)

Dosage Form

Capsules, each weighs 0.3 grams.

Dosage and Administration

Taken orally, 3 times daily, 4 capsules each time.

Effect

Replenishes *qi*, activates blood circulation, nourishes *yin*, supports *yang*, regulates menstruation, and treats leukorrhagia.

Indications

Irregular menstruation, dysmenorrhea, amenorrhea, leukorrhagia, sterility due to cold uterus, postpartum disorders, deficiency of vital essence due to consumption in male, and weakness of the loins and knees.

Manufacturer

Pharmaceutical Factory of Changchun College of Traditional Chinese Medicine and Dongfeng Pharmaceutical Factory in Jilin Province.

Notes

It is a newly developed medicine for women's healthcare.

2.3   Chinese Medicated Liquor for Healthcare

Chinese medicated liquors are a combination of liquor and traditional Chinese medicinal herbs that are used for healthcare. In ancient times, Chinese medicated liquors were called *Lao Li* or sweet wine with drugs. In the *Nei Jing*, there is a chapter entitled "On Lao Li," which gives a description of how the liquors were made and how they were used clinically. Since the Tang dynasty, medicated liquor has been extensively used in medical practice. With the development of both moral and material civilizations in China, medicated liquors, especially those for healthcare, were recorded in medical texts through the centuries. Even today these recipes are used to improve healthcare.

Medicated liquor is used for the treatment and prevention of diseases as well as for general healthcare. The majority of medicated liquors are used for nourishment, longevity, prophylaxis, and convalescence.

There are two types of medicated liquors: one for oral intake and the other for external application. They can be prepared in two ways.

- By steeping or boiling the herbs in Chinese white liquor, millet wine, or rice wine and then removing the herb residue from the medicated liquor.

- By putting a distiller's yeast into a mixture of herbs and cereal (polished glutinous rice or husked sorghum) and then fermenting the mixture. When the process is complete, the residue is then removed from the medicated liquor.

2.3.1   HEALTHCARE EFFECTS OF CHINESE MEDICATED LIQUOR

As a form of beverage, Chinese medicated liquor is convenient and can be taken over a long period of time. If chosen and taken properly, medicated liquor will exert the following benefits:

Regulating Yin and Yang

Good health and longevity is based on the harmony of *yin* and *yang* in the body. When this delicate balance is upset, illness and/or accelerated aging can set in. Chinese medicated liquor is good either for tonifying *yang,* nourishing *yin,* or both. Regular intake of a medicated liquor can help harmonize *yin* and *yang* and keep them in well dynamic equilibrium, thus maintaining health and longevity.

Invigorating Qi and Blood

Qi and blood are the vital material basis of life. *Qi* is reflected by the functional activities of the internal organs. The maintenance of the body's vital activities relies on the function of the body's *qi*. Deficiency of *qi* and blood will result in illness and quicken senility. It is recommended that who have those deficient *qi* and blood take medicated liquor, which is good for invigorating their *qi* and nourishing their blood. Taking medicated liquor will strengthen the body's resistance to diseases and slow down the process of senility.

Tonifying the Five Zang

The liver, heart, spleen, lungs, and kidneys transform and store nutritious substances such as vital essence, *qi*, blood, and body fluids.

As you grow and develop becoming strong or senile depends to a great extent on whether the physical function of the five *zang* organs are normal and whether their *qi*—especially the kidney-*qi*—is sufficient. Deficiency of the five *zang* organs is the cause of internal diseases and senility. Each of the five *Zang* organs performs its own functions. If an organ is deficient, symptoms and signs will manifest, and its deficiency can be detected. If proper medicated liquor is taken, the function of the dysfunctional organ can be restored to normal.

TCM theory explains that the kidneys are the origin of congenital constitution, while the spleen and stomach provide the material basis of the acquired constitution.

Among all the tonifying medicated liquors for healthcare, those that tonify the kidneys, aid the essential *qi*, and strengthen the spleen and stomach are most commonly seen and used. There are, however, medicated liquors that also tonify the heart and soothe the mind.

Eliminating Illness and Expelling Evils

In addition to various types of medicated liquors for tonification, there are also medicated liquors that are used for expelling wind, cold, and dampness; and for invigorating blood circulation by warming the channels and collaterals. These types of liquors are utilized in both the treatment of illnesses and for healthcare.

It is advisable for those suffering from *Bi* syndrome due to wind, cold or dampness, from hemiplegia caused by stroke, or from cardialgia caused by obstruction in the chest to take certain medicated liquors to aid in the recovery process.

Prolonging Life

Senility is caused when the *yin* and *yang* of the body is not properly harmonized, and when there is a deficiency in the five *zang* organs, an insufficiency of *qi* and blood, and/or the over-consumption of the essence of life. Tonic medicated liquors can delay the process of becoming senile. Taking such liquors frequently can makes strong bones, dark hair, smooth skin, and bright eyes so that one may enjoy health and longevity.

2.3.2 MECHANISM OF CHINESE MEDICATED LIQUOR

The active elements that compose Chinese medicated liquors are soluble in alcohol, which is the base material for the medicated liquors. It is the easy assimilation of the alcohol by the body that adds to the effectiveness of these medicated liquors. Thousands of years of clinical experience and research have shown that these commonly used liquors and their active principles play a part in preserving health and prolonging life. For example:

Ren Shen (*Radix ginseng*) is commonly used to help resist senility; it reinforces immunity, regulates internal secretions, promotes the synthesis of proteins, strengthens resistance to fatigue, resists myocardial ischemia, reduces blood sugar levels, and enhances the hematopoietic function.

Huang Qi (*Radix astragali*) prolongs the life of cells in vivo, reinforces immunity, strengthens muscle contractility and the capacity of stress reaction, promotes the synthesis of protein, dilates blood vessels, and decreases high blood pressure.

- *Ling Zhi* (*Ganoderma lucidum seu japonicum*) strengthens immunity and tolerance of oxygen deficiency, resists myocardial ischemia, and regulates the metabolism of nucleic acids.

- *Dang Gui* (*Radix angelicae sinensis*) increases the blood production, strengthens immunity, reinforces muscle contractility and body resistance to cold, protects the liver, increases the volume of blood flow in the heart muscles, resists myocardial ischemia and arrhythmia, hinders the accumulation of blood platelets to prevent thrombosis, and helps delay senility by means of anti-oxidation.

- *He Shou Wu* (*Radix polygoni multiflori*) resists atherosclerosis and myocardial ischernia, strengthens cellular immunity, checks lipid peroxide, and promotes the activity of diverged peroxidase to resist senility.

- *Gou Qi Zi* (*Fructus lycii*) decreases blood sugar and cholesterol levels, relieves atherosclerosis, and protects the liver.
- *Shan Zha* (*Fructus crataegi*) lowers high blood pressure and blood lipids, resists myocardial ischemia, and promotes digestion.
- *Ju Hua* (*Flos chrysanthemi*) increases the volume of blood flow in the coronary arteries, resists myocardial ischemia and thrombosis, and contains selenium (which is good for delaying the process of becoming senile).

These and other medicated liquors of TCM play an important role in healthcare because they help to protect the body against foreign pathogens and help to prolong life.

In recent years, experiments and research have been conducted on medicated liquors. Shanghai Medical Industry Institute conducted a study on *Shi Quan Da Bu Jiu* that reveals that this medicated liquor strengthens non-specific immunity, enhances gastrointestinal movement, increases the volume of blood flow in the coronary arteries, and reinforces the tolerance of oxygen deficiency. Such conclusions help explain in part why this medicated liquor is effective in invigorating *qi* and activating the functional activities of the spleen. Modern scientific investigation not only affirms the actions of medicated liquors, but it helps to reveal the mechanisms that lead to the correct utilization of the liquor.

2.3.3 CHARACTERISTICS OF HEALTHCARE WITH CHINESE MEDICATED LIQUOR

Liquor Helps the Effectiveness of Medicines

Liquor has the potency to promote blood circulation, resist cold, and make medicines potent. A saying in *Ben Cao Gang Mu* states: "By regulating *qi* and blood, proper drinking makes people vigorous and warm." Likewise, the book, *Ming Yi Bie Lu,* asserts, "Liquor helps spread the medicinal effect over the whole body." The nature of liquor is to warm up and regulate *qi* and blood. Liquor potentates medicine, dispels cold, and warms up and invigorates blood circulation. The main component of liquor is alcohol, an effective solvent that is apt to penetrate the tissues of crude drugs to dissolve certain elements in them. In crude medicinal materials, a lot of active elements such as alkaloids and their salts, volatile oils, glucosides, tannins, organic acids, resins, sugars, and some pigments can be easily dissolved in liquor. An experiment done with mice to compare the different immune effects of *Gui Ling Ji Jiu* and the crude or refined powder of *Gui Ling Ji* proved that the effect of *Gui Ling Ji Jiu* was much better.

Wide Indications and Easy Preparation

Medicated liquor is accepted widely in China. It makes healthy people stronger and free from illness. It helps the middle-aged and the elderly delay the process of aging. It serves as a supplementary treatment for patients with chronic diseases due to the imbalances of *yin* and *yang*, *qi* and blood, *zang* and *fu*, and it promotes the restoration of health. According to individual conditions, seasons, and sources of medicinal substances, a prescription of a medicated liquor may be easily readjusted and its preparation may be readily made.

Stable Effect and Convenient Administration

Liquor can also serve as a preservative. It can delay the hydrolysis of certain effective elements of medicines when its alcohol content is more than 40%. The herbal medicines often used to prepare medicated liquors are: *Long Yan (Arillus longan)*, *Shan Zha (Fructus crataegi)*, *Sang Shen (Fructus mori)*, *Gou Qi (Fructus lycii)*, *Yi Mi (Semen coicis)*, and *Ju Hua (Flos chrysanthemi)*. They can be taken as food or medicines. Most medicines chosen in medicated liquor are mild in nature, and they are quite safe when taken properly.

2.3.4 INDICATIONS OF CHINESE MEDICATED LIQUOR FOR HEALTHCARE

Indications of Medicated Liquor for Replenishing Qi

Symptoms of *qi* deficiency include lassitude, low voice, languor, weakness in the limbs, poor appetite, spontaneous sweating, pale and corpulent tongue (sometimes with teeth prints), and feeble pulse.

Indications of Medicated Liquor for Nourishing Blood

Symptoms of blood deficiency include pale or sallow complexion, dizziness, blurring of vision, darkness before the eyes when rising suddenly, pale lips and nails, numbness of the hands and feet, whitish tongue and thready pulse.

Indications of Medicated Liquor for Nourishing Yin

Symptoms of *yin* deficiency include heat in the palms, soles, and chest; afternoon fever; dryness in the mouth and throat; insomnia; dizziness; blurring of vision; night sweating; constipation; brown urine; reddish tongue or tongue with little coating; and a rapid pulse.

Indications of Medicated Liquor for Reinforcing Yang

Symptoms of *yang* deficiency include general or local intolerance of cold, cold limbs, edema of the face and feet, impotence, cold semen, frequent night urination, loose stools, watery urine, whitish and plump tongue with moist fur, and a faint pulse.

Indications of Medicated Liquor for Tonifying the Five Zang Organs

Symptoms of heart deficiency include palpitations, insomnia or dreaminess, amnesia, and a slow and weak pulse with regular intervals or a slow pulse with irregular intervals.

Symptoms of spleen deficiency include a poor appetite, abdominal distension after meals, a feeling of comfort from pressure on the abdomen, sallow complexion, feeble muscles, and loose stools.

Symptoms of lung deficiency include asthma and shortness of breath, prolonged cough, whitish sputum, and low resistance to colds.

Symptoms of kidney deficiency include soreness of the back, weakness of the legs and knees or pain in the heels, difficulty hearing, weakness of the teeth and hair, dripping after urination or incontinence of urine, retrogression of sexual function and sterility.

Indications of Medicated Liquor for Prolonging Life

This type of liquor is good for the middle-aged and the elderly. It will tonify the kidney, reinforce the spleen, and nourish the *qi* and blood.

Indications of Medicated Liquor for Preventing Diseases and Building up Health

Medicated liquor is often used in the prevention and supplementary treatment and rehabilitation of certain diseases.

Additionally, there are medicated liquors that are used for tonifying both the *qi* and the blood. Such tonics are suitable for the symptoms and signs of deficiency of both *qi* and blood. Medicated liquors are also used for reinforcing *yin* and *yang*, in cases of *yin* and *yang* deficiency.

2.3.5 PREPARATION OF MEDICATED LIQUOR

There is a variety of methods used for preparing medicated liquors; these include: cold-steeping, hot-steeping; brewing, percolating, and circular-heating. Cold- and hot-steeping are used mainly for making medicated liquors at home. Percolating and circular-heating are used in industrial manufacturing. Drug materials, processing, and implements (tools) play a key role in the preparation of high-quality medicated liquors.

Raw Materials

Liquor. When making a medicated liquor, it is important to choose a type of liquor, which is a solvent with its own medical effect. The most commonly used solvents are Chinese white liquor, millet wine, and yellow rice wine.

White liquor includes various types of hard liquors. It is prepared through distillation process and is 40%–60% alcohol. Medicated liquor made up of white liquor maintains its medicinal effects and is suitable for those fond of strong drinking.

Yellow rice wine is prepared through a fermentation process. Yellow rice wine contains less than 20% alcohol, glucose, malt sugar, and various amino acids. Medicated liquor prepared from millet wine or yellow rice wine is suitable for those who do not like drinking very much, like the elderly and those who are in poor health. Because of its low alcohol content, medicated liquor made from yellow rice wine cannot be kept very long, so you must take it as you prepare it.

Grape wine can also be used. It is also prepared through fermentation and its alcohol content is 7–8 percent.

Crude Medicines. Crude medicines selected for use in medicated liquors should be processed in conventional ways so as to ensure their medicinal action and reduce their side effects. It should be noted too that crude medicines should have their impurities removed and should be washed before use. It is preferable that they should be sliced or ground so as to widen their contacting surface with the liquor. It is inadvisable to crush them so small that the medicated liquor becomes turbid. In some instances, crystal sugar or honey is added into the liquor to improve its palatability.

Process

Cold-steeping. In order to cold-steep a medicated liquor, place the cut or broken crude medicines and the liquor (or wine) into a suitable container according to the prescribed amount. Wrap the crude medicines in a cloth bag to suspend them in the liquor.

Seal the container. Stir or agitate it once a day for seven days. After 15–20 days, filter it to obtain the clear liquid. This liquid can then be taken according to the proper dosage.

Hot-steeping. Hot-steeping is nearly the same as the cold-steeping process. Place ingredients and liquor in a glass container as above. Wrap the crude medicines in a cloth bag to suspend them in the liquor. Place the open container in a pot with water and heat it until the liquid surface in the container becomes foamy. Remove the container, seal it, and keep it for over half a month. When the time is complete, filter the medicated liquor to obtain a clear liquid.

Another method is to decoct the crude medicines. Heat the decoction until it becomes a concentrated extract. Place the extract into the liquor after it is cooled. Seal the container. Some days later, filter the mixed liquid to obtain the liquor. This method is not advisable for crude medicines containing aromatic and volatile elements.

Brewing. Soak glutinous rice, round-grained non-glutinous rice, or husked sorghum in water. Then steam it until it is cooked. Cool it to 30°C, add distiller's yeast and the prepared crude medicines or concentrated extract from decoction, mix them evenly, put the mixture into a suitable container, seal it, and keep it at room temperature for one-two weeks. Press the brewed mixture and filter the liquid. Pour the liquid into a container, which is to be heated to 75°C–80°C to kill harmful bacteria. The medicated liquor obtained by this method has a mild nature suitable to be taken by the elderly and the weak.

Implements (Tools)

The principle in selecting implements is to ensure that no chemical reactions should occur between the container and the medicinal substances. Pottery, porcelain, glass jars, bottles, or earthenware pots are commonly used. It is important that each container have a proper fitting lid. Do not use a metal container unless it is made from stainless steel.

2.3.6 CAUTIONS FOR TAKING MEDICATED LIQUOR

Correct Administration

TCM theory stresses that diagnosis and treatment be based on the differentiation of symptoms and signs; so does the administration of medicated liquor. Healing will be most effective when the correct medicated liquor is administered. This means one that suits an individuals specific constitution, the symptoms, and the signs as observed through differentiation of deficiency and excessiveness, cold and heat, *zang* and *fu*, *qi* and blood, and *yin* and *yang*. Any medicated liquor should be administered according to its therapeutic effect and indications. It is important to note that not everyone is fit for taking tonic liquor or longevity-enhancing liquor.

Contraindications and Dosage

Medicated liquor contains a certain amount of alcohol. Intake of small amounts of alcohol will do more good than harm. Researches show that small amount of liquor, less than 30 grams per day, helps lessen the chances of death caused by coronary heart disease. It is suggested that for safety, the amount of alcohol intake should be controlled to less than 45 grams per day. Prolonged heavy drinking will harm the liver, the heart, and the nervous system.

The hazards of overdrinking alcohol are widely discussed in the ancient Chinese medical texts. For example, the book, *Ben Cao Gang Mu*, states, "Light drinking leads to invigorating *qi* and blood, making one warm and in high spirits, dispelling sorrow and bringing about cheerfulness; while heavy drinking results in the impairment of essence, blood, and stomach and in the promotion of phlegm and fire. Indulgence in heavy drinking may cause one to be ill or degenerative and ruin his (or her) family. Are not these hazards terrible?" With this in mind, it is important to understand the dosages and contraindications of medicated liquors. Generally, medicated liquor is not advisable for those who suffer from liver diseases, severe heart diseases, cardiac insufficiency, peptic ulcer, active TB, chronic nephritis, chronic enteritis, or severe hypertension. They are also not suitable for children, pregnant or lactating women, and those who are allergic to alcohol. Additionally, medicated liquors may not be suitable for women to take during menstruation and for patients with excessive fire due to *yin* deficiency. The prescribed amount of medicated liquor should not be exceeded. Special care should be taken when consuming medicated liquor that is made from drastic or toxic drugs. Such dosages should begin with small amounts and gradually increase only when you are sure that no side effects will occur. Medicated liquor that is mild in nature can be taken in larger dosages. Larger dosages are also suitable for younger patients and those who are strong. Small dosages are for the elderly, weak, or mild cases.

Light drinkers should take small dosages or take medicated liquor made of yellow rice liquor or liquor with a small ratio of alcohol.

Other Precautions

Other precautions should also be considered when administering medicated liquor.

The administration of medicated liquor is associated with the seasons. It is proper to take medicated liquor warm in nature, especially the tonic type, in winter. If taking such tonics in the summer, the dosage should be reduced.

The time of administration of medicated liquors also varies with the location of the disease. If the disease is located above the diaphragm, then it should be taken after meals. If the disease is located below the diaphragm then the liquor should be taken before meals. If you are taking medicated liquor to nourish the heart and sooth the mind or for regulating menstruation, it is advisable to take it at night.

Medicated liquor should be stored hermetically in a cool and dry place.

2.3.7 COMMONLY USED MEDICATED LIQUOR

Since ancient times, there has been a large variety of medicated liquors. In this section, only the more common ones will be recommended. Most of the prescriptions are based on historical medical books or modern clinical reports. Some of them have been readjusted in light of the author's own experience.

MEDICATED LIQUOR FOR TONIFYING QI

REN SHEN JIU

Main Ingredients
Ren Shen (*Radix ginseng* in form of coarse power)   30 grams
Bai Jiu (Chinese white liquor)   500 grams
Process
Cold-steeping or hot-steeping
Dosage and Administration
Take twice daily, in the morning and evening, 10–15 ml. each time.
Effect
Tonifies *qi* and the spleen and lungs, promotes the production of body fluids, and soothes the mind.
Indications
Shortness of breath, lassitude, poor appetite, dizziness, palpitation, impairment of body fluid, spontaneous sweating, impotence, diabetes, all caused by *qi* deficiency.
When the liquor is finished, the residue may be steeped a second time in proper amount of white liquor. After a second time the residue may be eaten finally.

SHEN QI YI QI BU

Main Ingredients
Huang Qi (*Radix astragali*)   45 grams
Dang Shen (*Radix codonopsis*)   45 grams
Chen Pi (*Pericarpium citri reticulatae*)   9 grams
Da Zao (*Fructus jujubae*)   10 dates
Bai Jiu (Chinese white liquor)   1000 grams
Process
Cold-steeping or hot-steeping
Dosage and Administration
Take warm, twice daily, 10–20ml. each time, in the morning and evening.

Effect

Replenishes *qi*, invigorates the spleen, and induces appetite and digestion.

Indications

Syndrome due to *qi* deficiency, marked by lassitude, languor, and poor appetite.

Notes

This medicated liquor is mild in nature; it is not as potent as *Ren Shen Jiu*.

SAN SHENG JIU

Main Ingredients

Ren Shen (Radix ginseng)	21 grams
Shan Yao (Rhizoma dioscoreae)	21 grams
Bai Zhu (Rhizoma atractylodis macrocephalae)	21 grams
Bai Jiu (Chinese white liquor)	500 grams

Process

Cold-steeping or hot-steeping

Dosage and Administration

Take warm on an empty stomach, three times a day in the morning, at noon and in the evening, 10–20 ml. each time.

Effect

Tonifies primordial *qi* and strengthens the spleen and stomach.

Indicators

General debility, *qi* deficiency, lassitude, anorexia, sallow complexion, and emaciation.

Source

Sheng Ji Zong Lu

HUANG QI SHENG MAI JIU

Main Ingredients

Ren Shen (Radix ginseng)	30 grams
Huang Qi (Radix astragali)	60 grams
Mai Dong (Radix ophiopogonis)	18 grams
Wu Wei Zi (Fructus schisandrae)	12 grams
Bai Jiu (Chinese.white liquor)	1000 grams

Process

Cold-steeping or hot-steeping

Dosage and Administration

Take in the morning and evening, 10–20 ml. each time.

Effect

Tonifies primordial *qi* and nourishes *yin*. This tonic also promotes the production of body fluids and consolidates superficial resistance to perspiration.

Indications

Qi deficiency accompanied by impairment of the body fluid due to *yin* deficiency, such as *yin* deficiency of the heart and lungs marked by asthma, cough, spontaneous sweating, thirst, and reddened and dry tongue. Other indications include feeble pulse or promordial *qi* impaired by heat, spontaneous sweating, and thirst.

Notes

This prescription is based on the famous prescription of *Sheng Mai San*; *Huang Qi* is added to the famous prescription so as to enhance the effect of replenishing *qi* to consolidate superficial resistance.

CHANG SHENG GU BEN JIU

Main Ingredients

Ren Shen (Radix ginseng)	60 grams
Gou Qi Zi (Fructus lycii)	60 grams
Shan Yao (Rhizoma dioscoreae)	60 grams
Wu Wei Zi (Fructus schisandrae)	60 grams
Tian Dong (Radix asparagi)	60 grams
Mai Dong (Radix ophiopogonis)	60 grams
Sheng Di (Rhizoma rehmanniae)	60 grams
Shu Di (Rhizoma rehmanniae praeparata)	60 grams
Bai Jiu (Chinese white liquor)	1500 grams

Preparation

Cut the herbs into slices and put into a silk bag. Steep in the liquor within a container. Seal the container and heat it in water for half an hour. Next bury the container in the earth for a few days to expel the evil fire. Finally, filter the liquor.

Dosage and Administration

Take twice daily in the morning and evening, 10–20 ml. each time.

Effect

Replenishes *qi*, reinforces *yin*, nourishes the liver and kidneys.

Indications

Syndrome due to deficiency of both *qi* and *yin*, marked by lassitude, soreness, and weakness of the loins and legs; upset, dry mouth; dizziness; blurred vision; palpitations; and early graying of hair, etc.

Source

Shou Shi Bao Yuan

Notes

The homemade type of this liquor may have lower amounts of the herbs and liquor and is prepared using the cold-steeping or hot-steeping methods.

MEDICATED LIQUOR FOR NOURISHING BLOOD

E JIAO JIU

Main Ingredients

E Jiao (Colla corii asini)	75 grams
Huang Jiu (millet wine)	500 grams

Preparation

Cut *E Jiao* into small pieces and place in a container. Immerse the *E Jiao* in *Huang Jiu*. Place the container over mild heat, and continue to add the rest of the *Huang Jiu* to the container in small amounts until all the *E Jiao* is melted. Allow the liquor to cool, and place it in a bottle.

Dosage and Administration

Take warm, on an empty stomach three times daily, in the morning, at noon and in the evening, 20–30 ml. each time.

Effect

Tonifies blood, nourishes *yin*, arrests bleeding, clears away lung-heat, and moistens dryness.

Indications

Deficiency of *yin*-blood manifested as sallow complexion, dizziness, blurring of vision, palpitations, fidgeting, insomnia, and dry cough.

This wine can also used for women who have suffered such bleeding disorders as uterine bleeding, menorrhagia, vaginal bleeding during pregnancy, and bleeding after miscarriage.

LONG YAN SANG SHEN JIU

Main Ingredients

Long Yan Rou (Arillus longan)	30 grams
Sang Shen (Fructus mori)	30 grams
Bai Jiu (Chinese white liquor)	500 grams

Process

Cold-steeping

Dosage and Administration

Take twice daily in the morning and evening, 10–20 ml. each time.

Effect

Nourishes *yin* and blood, tonifies the heart and spleen, soothes the mind, and promotes the production of body fluids.

Indications

Deficiency of the blood, *yin*, heart, and kidneys. Such deficiency can be indicated by dizziness, blurred vision, palpitations, insomnia, poor appetite, lassitude, forgetfulness, and early graying of the hair.

Notes

Bai Jiu may be substituted for *Huang Jiu* (millet wine or yellow rice wine) when it is prepared by the cold-steeping method. It may also be prepared by brewing. In this case *Bai Jiu* is replaced with round-grained non-glutinous rice and distiller's yeast.

The ingredients *Long Yan Rou* and *Sang Shen* are both dried fruits. They tonify the heart and spleen and sooth the mind.

Main Ingredients

Ju Hua (Flos crysanthemi)	250 grams
Gou Qi Zi (Fructus lycii)	500 grams
Dang Gui (Radix angelicae sinensis)	250 grams
Long Yan Rou (Arillus longan)	1500 grams
Bai Jiu (Chinese white liquor)	15 kg.
Jiu Niang (fermented glutinous rice)	5 kg.

Process

Cold-steeping or hot-steeping

Dosage and Administration

Take twice daily, in the morning and evening, 10–20 ml. each time.

Effect

Nourishes blood and vital essence, tonifies the heart, spleen, liver and kidney, calms the mind, and improves eyesight.

Indications

Deficiency of blood and vital essence; weakness of the heart, spleen, liver and kidneys; sallow complexion; dizziness; blurring of vision and/or dim eyesight; palpitations; insomnia; general debility; and amnesia.

Source

Ji Yan Liang Fang and *Hui Zhi Tang Jing Yan Fang.*

Notes

This tonic is also called *Yang Sheng Jiu* and *Gui Yuan Qi Ju Jiu.* Its modification *Gui Yuan Xian Jiu* in the book, *Shi Jian Ben Cao*, consists of only *Dang Gui* and *Long Yan Rou*, which tonify the heart and blood.

Main Ingredients

Long Yan Rou (Arillus longan)	250 grams
Zhi Shou Wu (Radix polygoni multiflori praeparata)	250 grams
Ji Xue Teng (Cauhs spatholobi)	250 grams
Mi Jiu (millet wine)	1500 grams

Process

Cold-steeping

Dosage and Administration

Take twice daily in the morning and evenings, 10–20 ml. each time.

Effect

Nourishes blood and vital essence, tonifies the liver and kidney, invigorates the heart, calms the mind, activates blood circulation, and dredges the channels and collaterals.

Indications

Deficiency of the heart-blood, consumption of the liver and kidney, sallow complexion, dizziness, blurred vision, palpitations, insomnia, and early graying of hair.

Main Ingredients

E Jiao (Colla corii asim)	30 grams
Dang Gui (Radix angelicae sinensis)	30 grams
Ai Ye (Folium artemisiae argyi)	9 grams
Sheng Di (Radix rehnianniae)	15 grams
Chuan Xiong (Rhizoma chuanxiong)	15 grams
Bai Shao (Radix paeonlae alba)	21 grams
Gan Cao (Radix glycyrrhizae)	9 grams
Huang Jiu (millet wine or yellow rice wine)	250 grams

Preparation

Pour Huang Jiu into an earthen pot with 250 grams of warm boiled water and the other coarsely ground ingredients—except the E Jiao. Heat the pot over a mild fire until the contents boil. Cool the pot and filter the liquor. Pour the filtered liquor into a clean empty earthen pot. Place the small pieces of E Jiao into the pot and heat the pot over a medium heat. Continue to stir the contents until the E Jiao is completely melted. Once the E Jiao is melted, the liquor is prepared.

Dosage and Administration

For medical treatment, take the entire amount on an empty stomach, three times daily, in the morning, at noon and in the evening.

Effect

Nourishes the blood, promotes blood circulation, arrests bleeding, regulates menstruation, and prevents miscarriages.

Indications

Hypermenorrhea due to deficiency of blood and impairment of Chong and Ren channels, metrorrhagia, metrastaxis, uterine bleeding during pregnancy, excessive fetal movement, and postpartum continuous bleeding.

Source

Jin Kui Yao Lüe and Qian Jin Fang.

MEDICATED LIQUOR FOR NOURISHING YIN

Main Ingredients

Nü Zhen Zi (Fructus ligustri lucidi)	90 grams
Mi Jiu (millet wine)	500 grams

Process

Cold-steeping

Dosage and Administration

Take on an empty stomach, twice daily in the morning and evening, 20 ml. each time.

Effect

Nourishes yin-blood, tonifies the liver and kidneys, clears away heat of the deficiency type, strengthens the tendons and bones, darkens the hair, and improves eyesight.

Indications

Yin deficiency of the liver and kidney, dizziness, blurring of vision, dim eyesight, soreness and weakness of the loins and knees, weakness of the tendons and bones, and early graying of the hair.

Notes

The book, *Yi Bian*, says that this wine can also be used for prolonging life.

Main Ingredients

Tian Dong (Radix asparagi)	60 grams
Mai Dong (Radix ophiopogonis)	60 grams
Mi Jiu (millet wine)	500 grams

Process

Cold-steeping

Dosage and Administration

Take on an empty stomach, twice daily in the morning and evening, 20–30 ml. each time.

Effect

Nourishes *yin*, removes heat from the lungs, tonifies the kidneys, invigorates the stomach, clears away heart-fire, eliminates fidgeting, and promotes the production of body fluids.

Indications

Cough due to lung-dryness, thick sputum, hemoptysis, thirst due to deficiency of body fluid, fidgeting, and constipation.

Main Ingredients

Yin Er (Tremella)	30 grams
Xiang Gu (Lentinus hodes)	30 grams
Mi Jiu (Millet wine)	500 grams

Process

Hot-steeping with an adequate amount of crystal sugar

Dosage and Administration

Take on an empty stomach, three times daily in the morning, at noon, and in the evening, 20 ml. each time.

Effect

Nourishes *yin*, replenishes *qi*, moistens the lungs, and invigorates the stomach.

Indications

Because this tonic is mild, it is good for those that have general debility. It is also used to treat those with the syndrome of *yin* deficiency and weakened *qi*, and serves as an adjutant treatment for *yin* deficiency due to lung-heat, cough, hemoptysis, and tumors.

Notes

The extracts from *Bai Mu Er* and *Xiang Gu* promote immunity, aid in resisting cancer, and reduce blood-fat levels.

GOU QI YAO JIU

Main Ingredients

Shu Di Huang (Rhizoma rhemanniae praeparata)
Huang Jing (Rhizoma polygonati)
Bai He (Bulbus lilii)
Yuan Zhi (Radix polygalae)
Bai Jiu (Chinese white liquor)

Dosage and Administration

Take warm, 2–3 times daily, 10–15 ml. each time.

Effect

Nourishes the kidneys and benefits the liver.

Indications

Deficiency of the liver and kidneys, general debility, emaciation, soreness and weakness of the loins and legs, and insomnia.

Note

This liquor is only produced by pharmaceutical factories.

YANG SHEN GU BEN JIU

Main Ingredients

Xi Yang Shen (Radix panacis quinquefolii)	21 grams
Tian Dong (Radix asparagi)	30 grams
Mai Dong (Radix ophiopogonis)	30 grams
Sheng Di (Radix rehmanniae)	30 grams
Shu Di (Rhizoma rehmanniae praeparata)	30 grams
Bai Jiu (Chinese white liquor)	1500 grams

Process

Hot-steeping

Dosage and Administration

Take on an empty stomach, twice daily in the morning and evening, 10–20 ml. each time.

Effect

Nourishes *yin*, replenishes *qi*, and tonifies the vital essence and blood.

Indications

Syndromes due to consumption of *yin*, deficiency of *qi*, and exhaustion of vital essence. Such syndromes are indicated by emaciation, listlessness, hectic fever, fidgeting, dry mouth and throat, shortness of breath, dry cough, soreness and weakness of the loins and knees, sallow complexion, early graying of hair, and sterility due to the deficiency of essence.

Notes

This prescription is the modification of the prescription of *Ren Shen Gu Ben Wan* recorded in the book *Rui Zhu Tang Jiug Yan Fang*. In this modification, *Ren Shen* is replaced with *Xi Yang*

Shen for the purpose of strengthening the action of nourishing *yin*. The book considers *Ren Shen Gu Ben Wan* to have the effect of keeping hair black and the face bright and of prolonging life.

Main Ingredients

Tian Dong (Radix asparagi)	30 grams
Mai Dong (Radix ophiopogonis)	30 grams
Shu Di (Rhizoma rehmanniae praeparata)	30 grams
Sheng Di (Radix rehmanniae)	30 grams
Shan Yao (Rhizoma dioscoreae)	30 grams
Lian Zi Rou (Semen nelumbinis)	30 grams
Da Zao (Fructus jujubae)	30 grams
Jiu (liquor)	2500 grams

Process

Hot-steeping

Dosage and Administration

Take on an empty stomach, twice daily in the morning and evening, 20 ml. each time.

Effect

Nourishes *yin*-blood, invigorates the kidneys, and strengthens the spleen.

Indications

Syndrome due to deficiency of *yin*-essence and weakness of the spleen and kidneys as indicated by sallow complexion, early graying of the hair, dry mouth and throat, fidgeting, poor appetite, weak limbs, and lassitude.

Source

Wan Shi Jia Chuan Yang Sheng Si Yao

Notes

Compared to *Yang Shen Gu Ben Jiu*, this liquor has the stronger effect of invigorating the kidney and strengthening the spleen but the less strong effect of nourishing *yin* and replenishing *qi*.

Main Ingredients

Gou Qi Zi (Fructus lycii)	120 grams
Dang Gui (Radix angelicae sinensis)	60 grams
Shu Di (Rhizoma relimanniae praeparata)	180 grams
Bai Jiu or *Huang Jiu* (Chinese white liquor or yellow rice wine)	3000 grams

Process

Hot-steeping

Dosage and Administration

Take on an empty stomach, twice daily in the morning and evening, 20 ml. each time.

Effect

Nourishes *yin*, replenishes vital essence, enriches the blood, and tonifies the liver and kidneys.

Indications

Syndrome due to deficiency of *yin*, blood and vital essence indicated by dizziness, blurred vision, dim eyesight, soreness and weakness of the loins and knees, early graying of hair, emission, prospermia, and male-sterility.

Source

Hui Zhi Tang Jing Yan Fang

MEDICATED LIQUOR FOR SUPPORTING YANG

XIAN LING PI JIU

Main Ingredients

Yin Yang Huo (Herba epimedii)	60 grams
Bai Jiu or *Huang Jiu* (Chinese white liquor or yellow rice wine)	500 grams

Process

Cold-steeping

Dosage and Administration

Take on an empty stomach, twice daily in the morning and evening, 10–15 ml. each time.

Effect

Strengthens *yang*, invigorates the kidneys, tonifies the liver, enhance the tendons and bones, and dispels wind and dampness.

Indications

Syndrome due to deficiency of the kidney-*yang*, marked by impotence, female sterility, soreness and weakness of the loins and knees, aversion to cold, lassitude, numbness of the limbs, stiffness of the muscles and tendons, and rheumatic pain.

GE JIE JIU

Main Ingredients

Ge Jie (Gecko)	1 pair
Huang Jiu (millet or yellow rice wine)	1000 grams

Process

Cut *Ge Jie* without head and legs into small pieces and steep the pieces in *Huang Jiu*.

Dosage and Administration

Take on an empty stomach, twice daily in the morning and evening, 10–20 ml. each time.

Effect

Reinforces the kidney-*yang*, supplements the lung-*qi,* replenishes vital essence and blood, and relieves cough and asthma.

Indications

Impotence due to deficiency of the kidney-*yang*, asthma due to deficiency of the kidney, cough due to deficiency of the lungs and asthma, and cough due to consumption of the deficiency type, weakened *yang-qi* due to prolonged diseases, lassitude, and shortness of breath.

LU RONG JIU

Main Ingredients

Lu Rong (Cornu cervi pantotrichuni)	9 grams
Shan Yao (Rhizonia dioscoreae)	30 grams
Bai Jiu (Chinese white liquor)	500 grams

Process

Cold-steeping

Dosage and Administration

Take on an empty stomach, twice daily in the morning and evening, 10–15 ml. each time.

Effect

Supplements the kidney-*yang*, replenishes vital essence and blood, strengthens the tendons and bones, and regulates *Chong* and *Ren* channels.

Indications

Lassitude due to deficiency of *yang* and essence, weakness of the limbs, dizziness, blurred vision, deafness, amnesia, coldness and dampness of scrotum, emission, enuresis, thin leukorrhea, and sterility due to coldness in the womb.

Source

Pu Ji Fang

FU FANG LU RONG CHONG CAO JIU

Main Ingredients

Lu Rong (Cornu cervi pantotrichum)	6 grams
Dong Chong Xia Cao (Cordyceps)	30 grams
Gou Qi Zi (Fructus lycii)	30 grams
Bai Jiu (Chinese white liquor)	500 grams

Process

Cold-steeping

Dosage and Administration

Take on an empty stomach, twice daily in the morning and evening, 10–15 ml. each time.

Effect

Tonifies the lungs, liver, and kidneys; relieves asthma and coughs; and removes sputum.

Indications

Phlegm-retention, asthma, and cough due to deficiency of the lungs and kidney.

Main Ingredients

Yang Gao Wan (goat testis)	1 pair
Yin Yang Huo (Herba epimedii)	150 grams
Xian Mao (Rhizoma curculiginis)	150 grams
Gou Qi Zi (Fructus lycii)	150 grams
Tu Si Zi (Semen cuscutae)	150 grams
Bai Jiu (Chinese white liquor)	10 kg.

Process

Cold-steeping

Dosage and Administration

Take on an empty stomach, twice daily in the morning and evening, 10 ml. each time.

Effect

Enhances *yang*, tonifies the kidneys, invigorates the liver, and strengthens the tendons and bones.

Indications

General debility due to deficiency of *yang* deficiency of the liver and kidney, lassitude, aversion to cold, soreness and weakness of the loins and knees, weakness of the muscles and tendons, impotence, cold sperm, and sterility due to coldness in the womb.

Main Ingredients

Hai Gou Bian (Peniet testes callorhini)
Mei Lu Bian (Peniet testes cervi)
Guang Gou Bian (Peniet testes canini)
Ren Shen (Radix ginseng)
Lu Rong (Cornu cervi pantotrichurn)
Da Hai Ma (Hippocampus)
Ge Jie (Gecko)
Shang Rou Gui (Cortex cinnarnomi)
Shang Chen Xiang (Lignum aquilariae resinatum)
Fei Yang Qi Shi (Actinoliturn)
Wu Hua Long Gu (Os draconis)
Fu Pen Zi (Fructus rubi)
Bu Gu Zhi (Fructus psoraleae)
Tu Si Zi (Semen cuscutae)
Yin Yang Huo (Flerba epirnedii)
He Shou Wu (Radix polygoni multiflori)
Sang Piao Xiao (Oötheca mantidis)
Ba Ji Tian (Radix morindae officinalis)
Shan Yu Rou (Fructus corni)
Dan Pi (Cortex moutan)
Huang Qi (Radix astragali)
Niu Xi (Radix achyranthis bidentatae)
Qi Guo (Fructus lycii)

Sheng Di (Radix rehmanniae)
Shu Di (Rhizoma rehmanniae praeparata)
Huang Bai (Cortex phellodendri)
Chuan Jiao (Pericarpium zanthoxyli)
Hang Shao (Radix paeoniae alba)
Dang Gui (Radix angelicae sinensis)
Bai Zhu (Rhizoma atractylodis macrocephalae)
Yun Ling (Poria)
Rou Cong Rong (Herba cistanchis)
Ze Xie (Rhizoma alismatis)
Chang Pu (Rhizoma acori tatarinowii)
Xiao Hui Xiang (Fructus foeniculi)
Gan Song (Rhizoma nardostachyos)
Shan Yao (Rhizoma dioscoreae)
Du Zhong (Cortex eurornniae)
Yuan Zhi (Radix polygalae)
Gao Liang Jiu (Chinese white liquor made of sorghum)

Dosage and Administration
Taken orally, twice daily, 30 ml. each time.

Effect
Promotes the generation of vital essence, enriches the blood, strengthens the brain, and tonifies the kidneys.

Indications
General debility, early senility, soreness in the loins and back, dizziness due to anemia, spontaneous sweating, night sweating, pallor, palpitations, amnesia, aversion to cold, insomnia, and anorexia due to *qi* deficiency.

Manufacturer
Yantai Pharmaceutical Factory of Traditional Chinese Medicines in Shandong Province

Notes
Regular intake of this tonic can build up health, prevent disease, and prolong life.

DONG BEI SAN BAO JIU

Main Ingredients
Ren Shen (Radix ginseng)
Lu Rong (Cornu cervi pantotrichum)
Diao Bian (Peniet testes martes)

Dosage and Administration
Taken twice daily, 10–30 ml. each time.

Effect
Warms the kidneys, reinforces *yang*, replenishes *qi*, strengthens the brain.

Indications
Syndrome due to deficiency of the kidney-*yang*, marked by impotence, premature ejaculation, soreness and weakness of the loins and knees, and a cold and damp feeling of the scrotum.

Manufacturer
Jilin Pharmaceutical Factory of Traditional Chinese Medicines

Main Ingredients
Ren Shen (Radix ginseng)
Lu Rong (Cornu cervi pantotrichum)
Long Yan Rou (Arillus longan)
Chen Pi (Pericarpium citri reticulatae)
Gou Ji (Rhizoma cibotii)
Gou Qi Zi (Fructus lycii)
Bu Gu Zhi (Fructus psoraleae)
Huang Jing (Rhizoma polygonati)
Jin Ying Zi (Fructus rosae laevigatae)
Yin Yang Huo (Herba epimedii)
Dong Chong Xia Cao (Cordyceps)
Huai Niu Xi (Radix achyranthis bidentatae)
Ling Zhi (Ganoderma lucidum seu japonicum)
Dang Gui (Radix angelicae sinensis)
Fo Shou (Fructus citri sarcodactylis)
Que Nao (Sparrow brains)
Dosage and Administration
Taken 2–3 times daily, 9–15 ml. each time.
Effect
Warms the kidneys, reinforces *yang,* nourishes *qi* and blood.
Indications
General debility, lassitude, soreness and weakness of the loins and limbs, impotence, emission, and prospermia.
Manufacturer
Beijing Pharmaceutical Factory of Traditional Chinese Medicines

MEDICATED LIQUOR FOR TONIFYING BOTH QI AND BLOOD

Main Ingredients

Huang Qi (Radix astragali)	30 grams
Dang Shen (Radix codonopsis)	30 grams
Dang Gui (Radix angelicae sinensis)	30 grams
Long Yan Rou (Arillus longan)	30 grams
Sang Shen Zi (Fructus mori)	30 grams
Chen Pi (Pericarpium citri reticulatae)	9 grams
Bai Jiu or *Huang Jiu* (white liquor or millet wine)	1500 grams

Process
Hot or cold-steeping
Dosage and Administration
Take on an empty stomach, twice daily in the morning and evening, 10–20 ml. each time.

Effect

Replenishes *qi*, tonifies the blood, nourishes the heart, and strengthens the stomach.

Indications

Listlessness, sallow complexion, lassitude, shortness of breath, languor, dizziness, blurring of vision, palpitations, amnesia, and poor appetite.

BA ZHEN JIU

Main Ingredients

Ren Shen (Radix ginseng)	9 grams
Fu Ling (Poria)	21 grams
Bai Zhu (Rhizoma atractylodis macrocephalae)	21 grams
Dang Gui (Radix angelicae sinensis)	21 grams
Bai Shao (Radix paeoniae alba)	21 grams
Shu Di (Rhizoma rehmanitiae praeparata)	24 grams
Chuan Xiong (Rhizoma chuanxiong)	12 grams
Gan Cao (Radix glycyrrhizae)	9 grams
Sheng Jiang (Rhizoina zingiberis recens)	9 grams
Da Zao (Fructus jujubae)	10 dates
Bai Jiu or *Huang Jiu* (white liquor or millet wine)	3000 grams

Process

Hot-steeping

Dosage and Administration

Take on an empty stomach, twice daily in the morning and evening, 10–15 ml. each time.

Effect

Tonifies *qi* and blood, strengthens the spleen, and activates blood circulation.

Indications

Deficiency of the spleen and stomach, insufficiency of *qi* and blood, and consumption of the heart and lungs.

Notes

Dang Shen (*Radix codonopsis pilosulae*) may be used to replace *Ren Shen* at a dosage of 30 grams.

SHI QUAN DA BU JIU

Main Ingredients

Huang Qi (Radix Astragall)	45 grams
Dang Shen (Radix Codonopsis Pilosulae)	45 grams
Fu Ling (Poria)	30 grams
Bai Zhu (Rhizoma Atractylodis Macrocephalae)	30 grams
Shu Di (Rhizoma Rehmanniae Praeparata)	45 grams
Dang Gui (Radix Angelicae Sinensis)	30 grams
Bai Shao (Radix Paeoniae Alba)	30 grams
Chuan Xiong (Rhizoma Chuanxiong)	15 grams

Rou Gui (Cortex Cinnamomi)	15 grams
Gan Cao (Radix Glycyrrhizae)	15 grams
Bai Jiu (Chinese white liquor)	5000 grams

Process

Cold or hot-steeping

Dosage and Administration

Take on an empty stomach, twice daily in the morning and evening, 10–15 ml. each time.

Effect

This liquor is warm in nature; it has a strong tonifying effect.

Indications

Syndrome due to deficiency of *qi* and blood and with the symptoms of *yin*-cold type.

MEDICATED LIQUOR FOR TONIFYING YIN AND YANG

CHONG CAO JIU

Main Ingredients

Dong Chong Xia Cao (Cordyceps)	30 grams
Bai Jiu (Chinese white liquor)	500 grams

Process

Cold-steeping

Dosage and Administration

Take on an empty stomach, twice daily in the morning and evening, 10–20 ml. each time.

Effect

Tonifies not only the kidney-*yang* but also the lung-*yin.* Arrests bleeding, eliminates phlegm, and relieves asthma and cough.

Indications

General debility in the convalescence, listlessness, lassitude, poor appetite, or spontaneous sweating and aversion to cold, impotence, emission, soreness and weakness of the loins and knees, prolonged cough, asthma of deficiency type, and hemotysis due to consumptive diseases.

ER XIAN JIU

Main Ingredients

Xian Mao (Rhizoma curculiginis)	30 grams
Yin Yang Huo (Herba epimedii)	30 grams
Ba Ji Tian (Radix morindae officinalis)	30 grams
Dang Gui (Radix angelicae sinensis)	30 grams
Huang Bai (Cortex phellodendri)	21 grams
Zhi Mu (Rhizoma anemarrhenae)	30 grams
Bai Jiu (Chinese white liquor)	2000 grams

Process

Cold-steeping

Dosage and Administration

Take on an empty stomach, three times daily in the morning, at noon and in the evening, 10–20 ml. each time.

Effect

Tonifies kidney-*yang*, nourishes kidney-*yin*, clears away kidney-fire, regulates the *Chong* and *Ren* channels.

Indications

Climacteric hypertension, climacteric syndrome, irregular menstruation, amenorrhea, and deficiency of both *yin* and *yang*.

Main Ingredients

Shu Di (Rhizoma rehmanniae praeparata)	90 grams
Sheng Di (Radix rehmanniae)	90 grams
Zhi Shou Wu (Radix polygoni multiflori praeparata)	90 grams
Gou Qi Zi (Fructus lycii)	90 grams
Sha Yuan Zi (Semen astragah complanati)	90 grams
Lu Jiao Jiao (Colla cornus cervi)	90 grams
Dang Gui (Radix angelicae sinensis)	75 grams
Hu Tao Rou (Semen juglandis)	75 grams
Long Yan Rou (Arillus longan)	75 grams
Rou Cong Rong (Herba cistanchis)	60 grams
Bai Shao (Radix paeoniae alba)	60 grams
Ren Shen (Radix ginseng)	60 grams
Niu Xi (Radix achyranthis bidentatae)	60 grams
Bai Zhu (Rhizoma atractylodis macrocephalae)	60 grams
Yu Zhu (Phizoma polygonati odorati)	60 grams
Gui Ban Jiao (Colla carapacis et plastri testudinis)	60 grams
Bai Ju Hua (Flos chrysanthemi)	60 grams
Wu Jia Pi (Cortex acanthopanacis)	60 grams
Huang Qi (Radix astragali)	45 grams
Suo Yang (Herba cynomorii)	45 grams
Du Zhong (Cortex eucommiae)	45 grams
Di Gu Pi (Cortex lycii radicis)	45 grams
Dan Pi (Cortex moutan)	45 grams
Zhi Mu (Rhizoma anemarrhenae)	45 grams
Huang Bai (Cortex phellodendri)	30 grams
Rou Gui (Cortex cinnamomi)	30 grams

Preparation

Grind all of the above ingredients into a coarse powder and wrap them in a silk bag. Place the bag in a jar, and add 25–30 kg. of warm liquor. Seal the jar and let it stand for 15–20 days so that the herbs steep. Filter the liquor. The bag of herbs can be reused for a second batch of medicated liquor.

Dosage and Administration

Take warm on an empty stomach, twice daily in the morning and evening, 10–20 ml. each time.

Effect

Invigorates *yin*, reinforces *yang*, nourishes blood, replenishes vital essence, supplements *qi*, tonifies the five *zang*, and strengthens the tendons and bones.

Indications
Syndrome due to deficiency of both *yin* and *yang*.
Source
Lin Shi Huo Ren Lu Hui Bian

MEDICATED LIQUOR FOR TONIFYING THE FIVE ZANG

Medicated liquors used for tonifying the five *zang* organs can also be used to tonify and regulate *qi*, blood, and *yin* and *yang*.

FU LING JIU

Main Ingredients

Fu Ling (Poria)	60 grams
Bai Jiu (Chinese white liquor)	500 grams

Process
Cold-steeping
Dosage and Administration
Take on an empty stomach, three times daily, before breakfast, lunch and supper or before bed, 10–20 ml. each time.
Effect
Strengthens the spleen, restores *qi*, nourishes the heart, and calms the mind.
Indications
General debility due to deficiency of the spleen, anorexia, lassitude, muscular numbness, emaciation, palpitations, and insomnia.

SHEN XIAN YAO JIU WAN

Main Ingredients

Mu Xiang (Radix aucklandiae)	9 grams
Ding Xiang (Flos caryophylli)	6 grams
Tan Xiang (Lignum santali)	6 grams
Qian Cao (Radix rubiae)	6 grams
Sha Ren (Fructus aniomi)	15 grams
Hong Qu (Monascus purpureus went)	30 grams

Preparation
Grind the above ingredients into fine powder. Make the powder into boluses with honey, each weighing 9 grams. Steep 1–3 boluses in 500 grams of white liquor.
Dosage and Administration
Take in an appropriate amount each time.
Effect
Strengthens the spleen, stops upward adverse flow of lung- or stomach-*qi*, promotes digestion, and relieves stuffiness of the chest.
Indications
Weakness of the spleen and stomach, anorexia, and fullness in the stomach after meals.

Source

The book *Qing Tai Yi Yuan Pei Fang*

YANG XIN AN SHEN JIU

Main Ingredients

Long Yan Rou (Arillus longan)	30 grams
Suan Zao Ren (Semen ziziphi spinosae)	30 grams
Fu Shen (Poria cum ligno hospite)	30 grams
Bai Zi Ren (Semen biotae)	15 grams
Wu Wei Zi (Fructus schisandrae)	15 grams
Mai Dong (Radix ophiopogonis)	15 grams
Bai Jiu (Chinese white liquor)	2000 grams

Process

Cold-steeping

Dosage and Administration

Take three times daily, 10 ml. in the morning and at noon, 20 ml. before bed.

Effect

Nourishes the heart, calms the mind, and enriches and tonifies the blood.

Indications

Palpitations, irritability, insomnia, lassitude, amnesia, deficiency of *yin*-blood and weakness of the heart and mind.

SHEN GE CHONG CAO JIU

Main Ingredients

Ren Shen (Radix ginseng)	30 grams
Ge Jie (Gecko with the head and legs removed)	a pair
Dong Chong Xia Cao (Cordyceps)	30 grams
Hu Tao Ren (Semen juglandis)	30 grams
Bai Jiu (Chinese white liquor)	2 kg.

Process

Cold-steeping

Dosage and Administration

Take warm on an empty stomach, twice daily in the morning and evening, 10–20 ml. each time.

Effect

Tonifies the lungs and kidneys, reinforces *yang-qi*, supplements vital essence and blood, and relieves asthma.

Indications

Deficiency and weakness of *yang-qi*, general debility due to prolonged disease, listlessness, lassitude, amnesia, insomnia, soreness and weakness of the loins and knees, asthma, and cough of the deficiency type.

Main Ingredients

Hai Ma (Hippocampus)	a pair
Ming Xia (shrimp)	30 grams
Yin Yang Huo (Herba epimedii)	15 grams
Bai Jiu (Chinese white liquor)	500 grams

Process
Hot or cold-steeping

Dosage and Administration
Take twice daily in the morning and evening, 10–20 ml. each time.

Effect
Tonifies the kidneys, supports *yang*, strengthens the tendons and bones, promotes digestion, and regulates *qi*.

Indications
Impotence due to deficiency of the kidney-*yang*, listlessness, lassitude, shortness of breath, soreness and weakness of the loins and knees, and frequent night-urination.

Main Ingredients

He Shou Wu (Radix polygoni multiflori)	30 grams
Gou Qi Zi (Fructus lycii)	30 grams
Ju Hua (Flos chrysanthemi)	30 grams
Dang Gui (Radix angelicae sinensis)	21 grams
Long Yan Rou (Arillus longan)	21 grams
Hu Ma Ren (Semen canabis)	30 grams
Bai Jiu (Chinese white liquor)	2000 grams

Process
Hot or cold-steeping

Dosage and Administration
Take twice daily in the morning and evening, on an empty stomach, 10–20 ml. each time.

Effect
Tonifies and nourishes the liver, kidneys, vital essence blood, improves eyesight, calms the mind, and slows down the process of aging.

Indications
Dizziness, blurring of vision, dim eyesight, listlessness, weakness of the loins and knees, early graying of hair, emission, leukorrhea, amnesia, palpitations (all due to deficiency of the liver, kidneys, vital essence, and blood).

Main Ingredients

Tian Dong (Radly asparagi)	120 grams
Mai Dong (Radix ophiopogonis)	120 grams

Sheng Di (Radix rehmanniae)	250 grams
Shu Di (Rhizoma rehmanniae praeparata)	250 grams
Ren Shen (Radix ginseng)	60 grams
Fu Ling (Poria)	60 grams
Gou Qi Zi (Fructus lycii)	60 grams
Sha Ren (Fructus arnomi)	21 grams
Mu Xiang (Radix aucklandiae)	15 grams
Chen Xiang (Lignum aquilariae resinaturn)	9 grams

Preparation

Grind the above ingredients into a coarse powder and put into a silk bag. Place the bag in a porcelain jar with 15 kg. of white liquor. Boil the jar in water until the liquor boils. Reduce the heat to medium for 30 minutes until the liquor turns dark. Allow the jar to cool and let it stand for a few days. Finally, remove the liquor for use.

Dosage and Administration

Take on an empty stomach, twice daily in the morning and evening, 10–20 ml. each time.

Effect

Invigorates qi, tonifies the blood, nourishes yin, regulates and supplements the five organs, strengthens the stomach, and promotes the flow of qi.

Indications

Listlessness, pale complexion, lassitude, languor with no desire for speaking, early graying of hair, dizziness, blurring of vision, weakness of the loins and knees, poor appetite, amnesia, palpitation, etc. (all due to weakness of the five zang and deficiency of qi and blood).

MEDICATED LIQUOR FOR PROLONGING LIFE

This type of medicated liquor is used to delay aging by harmonizing yin and yang, tonifying qi and wood, and nourishing the five zang organs. Some of the liquors introduced above, if they taken regularly, are also effective in slowing down the process of becoming senile.

The following are medicated liquors that are used to prolong life.

BAI SUI HU

Main Ingredients

Mi Zhi Huang Qi (honeyed radix astragali)	60 grams
Fu Shen (Poria cum ligno hospite)	60 grams
Dang Gui (Radix angelicae sinensis)	36 grams
Shu Di (Rhizoma rehmanniae praeparata)	36 grams
Sheng Di (Radix rehmanniae)	36 grams
Dang Shen (Radix codonopsis)	30 grams
Mai Dong (Radix ophiopogonis)	30 grams
Fu Ling (Poria)	30 grams
Bai Zhu (Rhizoma atractylodis macrocephalae)	30 grams
Zao Pi (Fructus corni)	30 grams

Chuan Xiong (Rhizoina chuanxiong)	30 grams
Gui Ban Jiao (Colla carapacis et plastri testudinis)	30 grams
Fang Feng (Radix saposhinkoviae)	30 grams
Gou Qi (Fructus lycii)	30 grams
Chen Pi (Pericarpium citri reticulatae)	30 grams
Wu Wei Zi (Fructus schisandrae)	24 grams
Qiang Huo (Rhizoma seu radix notopterygii)	24 grams
Rou Gui (Cortex cinnarnomi)	18 grams
Hong Zao (Fructus jujubae)	1000 grams
Bing Tang (crystal sugar)	1000 grams
Gao Liang Jiu (sorghum liquor)	10 kg.

Preparation

Place the above ingredients into a porcelain pot and boil for about two hours. Bury the pot in earth for seven days. Unearth the pot and filter the liquor for use.

Dosage and Administration

Take as pre-prescribed amount.

Effect

Tonifies the *qi* and blood, nourishes *yin*-essence, strengthens the kidney-fire, promotes the flow of *qi*, dispels wind, reinforces the five *zang* organs, blackens hair, brightens the face, and prolongs life.

Indications

Deafness, decline of eyesight, grey hair, pale complexion, and weakness.

Source

Yao Fang Za Lu

YAN SHOU JIU XIAN JIU

Main Ingredients

Ren Shen (Radix ginseng)	60 grams
Chao Bai Zhu (parched *Rhizoma atractylodis macrocephalae*)	60 grams
Fu Ling (Poria)	60 grams
Chao Gan Cao (Parched *radix glycyrrhizae*)	60 grams
Dang Gui (Radix Angelicae sinensis)	60 grams
Chuan Xiong (Rhizonia chuanxiong)	60 grams
Shu Di (Rhizoma rehmanniae praeparata)	60 grams
Chao Bai Shao (Radix paeoniae alba parched with liquor)	60 grams
Gou Qi Zi (Fructus lycii)	250 grams
Sheng Jiang (Rhizoma zingiberis recens)	60 grams
Da Zao (Fructus jujubae with the core removed)	30 dates
Bai Jiu (Chinese white liquor)	17.5 kg.

Process

Hot-steeping

Dosage and Administration

Take as prescribed.

Effect

Tonifies the *qi* and blood and invigorates the liver and kidneys.

Indications

Deficiency of *qi* and blood and weakness of the liver and kidney.

Source

Ming Yi Xuan Yao Ji Shi Qi Fang

LIAO BAI JI YAN SHOU JIU

Main Ingredients

Huang Jing (Rhizoma polygonati)	60 grams
Tian Dong (Radix asparagi)	45 grams
Song Ye (Folium pini)	90 grams
Cang Zhu (Rhizoma atractylodis)	60 grams
Gou Qi Zi (Fructus lycii)	75 grams
Bai Jiu (Chinese white liquor)	5 kg.

Dosage and Administration

Take twice daily in the morning and evening, 10–20 ml. each time.

Effect

Nourishes the kidneys, moistens the lungs, replenishes the liver, tonifies the spleen, enriches *yin*-essence, invigorates the heart-*qi*, improves eyesight, removes wind and dampness, and strengthens tendons and bones.

Indications

Lassitude, decline of appetite, dizziness, dim eyesight, stiff muscles and joints, restlessness, insomnia, and early graying of hair.

Source

Zhong Zang Jing

JING SHEN YAO JIU

Main Ingredients

Ren Shen (Radix ginseng)	15 grams
Sheng Di (Radix rehmarmiae)	15 grams
Gou Qi Zi (Fructus lycii)	15 grams
Yin Yang Huo (Herba epimedii)	9 grams
Sha Yuan Zi (Semen astragali complanati)	9 grams
Mu Ding Xiang (Fructus eugenia caryophyllata)	9 grams
Chen Xiang (Lignum aquilariae resinatum)	3 grams
Yuan Zhi Rou (Radix polygalae)	3 grams
Li Zhi He (Semen litchi)	7 pieces
Gao Liang Jiu (sorghum liquor)	1 kg.

Process

Cold-steeping for 45 days

Dosage and Administration

Take 10 ml. once a day.

Effect

Replenishes *qi*, reinforces *yang*, nourishes *yin*, invigorates the liver and kidneys, strengthens the spleen and stomach, calms the mind, improves intelligence, dispels cold, relieves pain, restores energy, and slows down the aging process.

Notes

This medicated liquor was developed by the famous contemporary TCM physician, Wu Zhaoxian. It was introduced to the Sichuan Journal of TCM by his student.

MEDICATED LIQUOR FOR PREVENTING DISEASES

The following medicated liquors are commonly used in the prevention of disease.

JU ZHA YI XIN JIU

Main Ingredients

Ju Hua (Flos chrysanthemi)	30 grams
Shan Zha (Fructus crataegi)	45 grams
Bai Jiu (Chinese white liquor)	500 grams

Process

Cold-steeping

Dosage and Administration

Taken three times daily, 10–20 ml. each time.

Effect

Calms the liver, improves eyesight, expels wind, removes heat, strengthens the stomach, promotes digestion, and dissipates stasis. Additionally, this liquor is suitable for the prevention and treatment of coronary heart disease.

Indications

Hypertension, hyperlipemia, and atherosclerosis.

JIAN XIN LING JIU

Main Ingredients

Huang Qi (Radix astragali)	30 grams
Dan Shen (Radix salviae miltiorrhizae)	30 grams
Chuan Xiong (Rhizoma chuanxiong)	12 grams
Gui Zhi (Ramulus cinnamomi)	6 grams
Bai Jiu (Chinese white liquor)	500 grams

Process

Cold-steeping

Dosage and Administration

Take three times daily, 10–20 ml. each time.

Effect

Replenishes *qi*, activates blood circulation, induces the flow of *yang*, strengthens resistance to fatigue, and enhances hypoxia tolerance.

Indications

This tonic is suitable for the prevention and treatment of coronary heart disease and ischemic cerebrovascular disease.

Notes
This tonic was developed by the Affiliated Hospital of Shandong College of Traditional Chinese Medicine

TU SU JIU

Main Ingredients
Ma Huang (Herba ephedrae)
Chuan Jiao (Pericarpium zanthoxyli)
Xi Xin (Herba asari)
Fang Feng (Radix saposhinkoviae)
Cang Zhu (Rhizoma atractylodis)
Gan Jiang (Rhizoma zingiberis)
Rou Gui (Cortex cinnamomi)
Jie Geng (Radix platycodi)

Preparation
Grind the above ingredients into a coarse powder. Place the powder in a silk bag. Steep the bag in an adequate amount of white liquor within a container. Seal the container and let it stand for three days. Then filter out the liquor for use.

Dosage and Administration
Take according to prescribed amount.

Effect
Expels wind, disperses cold, and warms the middle *jiao* to strengthen the spleen.

Indications
Prevention and treatment of common cold due to wind-cold and stomachache due to cold.

Source
Jing Yue Quan Shu (Jing Yue's Complete Works)

Notes
This is a medicated liquor traditionally used in China for the prevention of infectious epidemic diseases. There are many prescriptions for this liquor, some of which contain toxic or excessively potent drugs. Such prescriptions are not introduced here; however, it must be pointed out that they must be taken with great care.

DU HUO JI SHENG JIU

Main Ingredients

Sheng Di (Radix relinianniae)	9 grams
Bai Shao (Radix paeoniae alba)	9 grams
GuiYin (Ramulus cinnamomi)	9 grams
Fu Ling (Poria)	9 grams
Du Zhong (Cortex eucominiae)	9 grams
Niu Xi (Radix achyranthis bidentatae)	9 grams
Sang Ji Sheng (Ramulus lorandii)	15 grams
Du Huo (Radix Angelicae pubesceills)	6 grams

Qin Jiao (Radix Gentianae macrophyllae)	6 grams
Chuan Xiong (Rhizonia chuanxiong)	6 grams
Ren Shen (Radix ginseng)	6 grams
Fang Feng (Radix Saposfiinkoviae)	6 grams
Xi Xin (Herba Asari)	3 grams
Dang Gui (Radix Angelicae Sineasis)	3 grams
Gan Cao (Radix Glycyrrhizae)	3 grams
Bai Jiu (Chinese white liquor)	1000 grams

Process

Cold-steeping

Dosage and Administration

Taken 1–2 times daily, 20–30 ml. each time.

Effect

Tonifies the liver and kidneys, replenishes *qi* and blood, dispels wind and dampness, and relieves rheumatic pain.

Indications

Weakness of the liver and kidneys and deficiency of *qi* and blood, indicated by rheumatoid arthritis, chronic pain of the loins and legs, and sciatica.

This tonic is also suitable for the treatment of the syndromes of wind, cold, and dampness due to weakness of the liver and kidneys and deficiency of *qi* and blood.

Source

Wan Bing Hui Chun

Notes

This medicated liquor can strengthen the body's resistance and help to eliminate pathogenic factors.

SHEN RONG JIU

Main Ingredients

Ren Shen (Radix ginseng)	60 grams
Lu Rong (Cornu cervi pantotrichum)	30 grams
Dang Gui (Radix angelicae sinensis)	6 grams
Qin Jiao (Radix gentianae macrophyllae)	6 grams
Hong Hua (Flos carthami)	6 grams
Gou Qi Zi (Fructus lycii)	6 grams
Fang Feng (Radix saposhinkoviae)	3 grams
Bie Jia (Carapax trionycis)	3 grams
Bi Xie (Rhizoma dioscroreae hypoglaucae)	3 grams
Qiang Huo (Rhizoma seu radix notopterygii)	3 grams
Chuan Niu Xi (Radix achyranthis bidentatae)	3 grams
Du Huo (Radix angelicae pubescentis)	3 grams
Du Zhong (Radix eucommiae)	3 grams
Bai Zhu (Rhizoma atractylodis macrocephalae)	3 grams
Yu Zhu (Rhizoma polygonati odorati)	3 grams
Ding Xiang (Flos caryophylli)	2.4 grams

Preparation
Place in a container the above ingredients and 10 kg. of white liquor that has been stored for many years. Seal the container and let it stand for several years. Filter the liquor and add 120 grams of crystal sugar and 1 kg. of white liquor to it. The medicated liquor is now ready to be taken.
Dosage and Administration
Take twice daily, 10–20 ml. each time.
Effect
Replenishes *qi* and warms *yang*. It also tonifies the liver and kidneys, nourishes *yin*-essence, strengthens the loins and knees, dispels wind, removes dampness, and activates blood circulation.
Indications
This tonic can be used to treat all disorders due to the invasion of wind, to cold or damp evils and to those that reflect deficiency of *qi* and blood and weakness of the liver and kidneys.
Source
Qing Tai Yi Yuan Pei Fang

2.4 Soft Extracts

A soft extract is a thick, viscous preparation of decocted herbal medicines in water and thickened with sugar or honey. Such medicine has been prepared and used since ancient times. Today, these extracts are still regarded as effective patent medicines. In southern China, soft extracts are regarded as a good tonic to be taken during the winter months.

Soft extracts have been used in the prevention and treatment of various kinds of diseases. They are mild and have long-term potency, are convenient to store, and simple to prepare. Soft extracts are an economical and practical medicine for healthcare.

Soft extracts are usually made up of many ingredients. Their composition and applications are based on differentiation of many concerned factors. They can strengthen and adjust the whole body consolidating the constitution and slowing down the process of aging by regulating *yin* and *yang*, enriching *qi* and blood, nourishing the five *zang* organs, and supplementing vital essence and marrow. They also build up the body by eliminating evil factors, preventing certain diseases, and restoring health.

Soft extracts are usually taken with warm boiled water. They can be taken in various ways in order to meet the specific need of a patient.
- Some are sucked in the mouth (to treat throat disorders)
- Some (for tonification) are taken on an empty stomach

- Some (for nourishing the liver or to calm the mind) are taken before bedtime
- Some are taken half an hour before meals (to treat diseases in the lower *jiao*)
- Some are taken half an hour after meals (to treat diseases in the upper *jiao*)

The dosage of soft extracts is determined according to the nature of the ingredients, the disease condition, and the patient's constitution. Mild-natured soft extracts without toxicity, especially those made of edible medicines, may be taken in larger dosage. Soft extract containing potent or toxic ingredients should be taken in small dosages. When first taking a soft extract, it is wise to start with a small dosage and then gradually increase it when you are sure that there will be no side effects. The dosages of the following prescriptions are those prescribed for adults. They may be modified to a certain extent depending on the constitution of the patient.

Following are the usual methods for making at home soft extracts for healthcare.

Preparation of Materials. Prepare all of the ingredients as follows: Remove dust and impurities from the herbal medicines and process them according to the prescription. White, granulated, or crystal sugar is usually used; brown sugar is used in rare occasions. The sugar is processed, by either parching or melting. To parch sugar, place it into a bronze pot and heat until the sugar is melted; the color will become yellowish, and bubbles and whitish smoke will appear. When you are parching sugar, stir frequently so that the sugar heats evenly.

To melt sugar, follow the following steps. Place 10 kg. of sugar and 5–6 kg. of water in a pot and boil together for half an hour or so. Add the prescribed amount of 10% tartaric acid while stirring. Continue to boil for two hours. This process transforms the glucose in the cane sugar into fructose.

Honey can also be used in making soft extracts. To prepare the honey, heat it in a pot until it is melted, remove the foam, which will allow nearly all the water in the honey to evaporate. When the color becomes brown and large bubbles appear, add water, equal to 10% of the heated honey. Maintain the heat until the contents boil. Filter the contents while they are still hot to remove impurities; pour out the contents from the pot while still hot, and filter it with a silk sifter to remove the impurities.

Concentration and Decoction. Decoct the medicines in water for a few hours. Allow them to steep for up to five hours.

Repeat this process twice. Filter out the residue and squeeze the juice out of it. Combine the decoction and the juice, and let the mixture settle. Filter the mixture with layers of gauze and heat it once again until it boils. Remove the surface foam and continue to simmer the decoction slowly. It is important to continue to stir the decoction as it cooks down so as to prevent sticking or burning. Continue this process until the decoction is thick and viscous.

Preparation of Soft Extract. Combine equal amounts of processed sugar or honey with the concentrated decoction. This completes the preparation of the soft extract. Be sure not to use an iron pot when preparing a soft extract.

Storage. Soft extracts are stored in a glass, enamel, pottery, or porcelain containers and kept airtight in a cool, dark place.

The following are various types of soft extracts that are commonly used for healthcare. The dosages, preparations, and analyses of effects are enriched by the author's modern knowledge and experience. Prescriptions without sources indicated have been established by the author.

2.4.1 SOFT EXTRACTS FOR INVIGORATING *QI*

REN SHEN GAO

Main Ingredients

Ren Shen (Radix ginseng)	250 grams

Preparation

Crush *Ren Shen* into a coarse powder and decoct it three times. Condense the decoctions, and add the refined honey to produce the extract.

Dosage and Administration

Take twice daily, in the morning and evening, 15 grams each time.

Effect

Enriches the primordial *qi*, strengthens the spleen, enhances mental power, and prevents senility.

Indications

Syndromes due to deficiency of *qi* and infirmity with age.

Source

Jing Yue Quan Shu

DAI SHEN GAO

Main Ingredients

Dang Shen (Radix codonopsis)	250 grams
Huang Qi (Radix astragali)	250 grams
Bai Zhu (Rhizoma atractylodis macrocephalae)	250 grams
Long Yan Rou (Arillus longan)	250 grams

Preparation

Decoct the above ingredients. Condense the decoction and add 250 grams of processed sugar.

Dosage and Administration

Take twice daily in the morning and evening, 15 grams each time.

Effect

Replenishes *qi*, strengthens the spleen, and nourishes the heart.

Indications

Syndromes due to deficiency of *qi*, general debility, and *qi* deficiency of the heart and spleen in particular.

Source

Zhong Yao Cheng Fang Pei Ben

YI QI KAI WEI GAO

Main Ingredients

Ren Shen (Radix ginseng)	30 grams
Fu Ling (Poria)	250 grams
Huang Qi (Radix astragali)	250 grams
Chao Mai Ya (parched *Fructus hordei germinatus*)	250 grams
Shan Zha (Fructus crataegi)	250 grams
Sha Ren (Fructus amomi)	15 grams

Preparation

Decoct the above ingredients. Condense the decoction, and add the prescribed amount of refined honey.

Dosage and Administration

Take twice daily in the morning and evening, 15 grams each time.

Effect

Replenishes *qi*, strengthens the spleen, and removes undigested food. It also promotes the flow of *qi* and activates the functional activities of the stomach.

Indications

General debility, *qi* deficiency, weakness of the spleen and stomach, and poor appetite.

Notes

This extract can exert both tonifying and resolving actions at the same time.

2.4.2 SOFT EXTRACTS FOR NOURISHING THE BLOOD

SANG SHEN GAO

Main Ingredients

Sang Shen (Fructus Mori)	1000 grams

Preparation

Pound and squeeze *Sang Shen* to get its juice. Condense the juice and add an adequate amount of refined honey to form the extract.

Dosage and Administration

Take 2–3 times daily, 30 grams each time.

Effect

Nourishes the blood and *yin*, darkens hair, and moistens the large intestine.

Indications

Early graying of hair, constipation due to dryness in the intestines, and deficiency of *yin*-blood.

Source

Su Wen Bing Ji Qi Yi Bao Ming Ji

QI YUAN GAO

Main Ingredients

Gou Qi Zi (Fructus lycii)	500 grams
Long Yan Rou (Arillus longan)	500 grams

Preparation

Decoct the above ingredients. Condense the extract and add an adequate amount of refined honey.

Dosage and Administration

Take 2–3 times daily, 15–30 grams each time.

Effect

Supplements the vital essence and blood, nourishes the heart, calms the mind, and invigorates the liver and kidneys.

Indications

Insufficiency of the heart-blood and weakness of the liver and kidneys.

Source

The book *She Sheng Mi Zhi*

Notes

This extract can also calm the mind, nourish Wood, strengthen tendons and bones, moisten muscles and skin, and brighten the complexion.

SHOU WU BU XUE GAO

Main Ingredients

He Shou Wu (Radix pollygoni multiflori)	250 grams
Da Zao (Fructus jujubae)	500 grams
Sang Shen Zi (Fructus mori)	500 grams
Long Yan Rou (Arillus longan)	500 grams
Hei Zhi Ma (Semen sesami nigrum)	500 grams

Preparation

Decoct the above ingredients. Condense the decoction and add an adequate amount of refined honey.

Dosage and Administration

Take 2–3 times daily, 15–30 grams each time.

Effect

Nourishes the blood, invigorates *qi* and *yin*, enhances the heart and spleen, darkens the hair, and moistens the large intestine.

Indications

Insufficiency of *yin*-blood, early graying of hair, dysphoria, and constipation due to dryness in the intestines.

Notes

This extract is a mild tonic for enriching *yin*-blood. It will also moisten muscles and skin and brighten the complexion.

DANG GUI BU XUE GAO

Main Ingredients

Dang Gui (Radix angelicae sinensis)
Chuan Xiong (Rhizoma chuanxiong)
Huang Qi (Radix astragali)
Gan Cao (Radix glycyrrhizae)
Dang Shen (Radix codonopsis)
Bai Shao (Radix paeoniae alba)
E Jiao (Colla corii asini)
Fu Ling (Poria)
Shu Di (Rhizoma rehmanniae praeparata)

Dosage and Administration

Take according to the instructions.

Effect

Nourishes the blood and replenishes *qi*.

Indications

General debility, sallow complexion, dizziness, blurred vision, deficiency of blood, and consumption of blood after giving birth.

Manufacturer

Zhonglian Pharmaceutical Factory in Wuhan City

2.4.3 SOFT EXTRACT FOR NOURISHING *YIN*

ER DONG GAO

Main Ingredients

Tian Dong (Radix asparagi)	500 grams
Mai Dong (Radix ophiopogonis)	500 grams

Preparation

Decoct the above ingredients. Condense the decoction and add an adequate amount of refined honey.

Dosage and Administration

Take 2-3 times daily, 15 grams each time.

Effect

Nourishes *yin*, moistens the lungs, and expels fire.

Indications

Consumption of body fluid due to *yin* deficiency, cough due to phlegm-heat, lung-dryness due to *yin* deficiency in the middle-aged and elderly.

Source

Zhang Shi Yi Tong

ER ZHI GAO

Main Ingredients

Nu Zhen Zi (Fructus ligustri lucidi)	500 grams
Han Lian Cao (Herba ecliptae)	500 grams

Preparation

Decoct the above ingredients. Condense the decoction and add an adequate amount of refined honey.

Dosage and Administration

Take 2–3 times daily, 15 grams each time.

Effect

Nourishes *yin*, invigorates the kidneys, and enhances the liver.

Indications

Syndrome due to *yin* deficiency of the liver and kidneys, marked by dizziness, tinnitus, insomnia, early graying of hair, soreness of the loins and knees, emission, night sweating, and hemorrhage.

Source

Yang Shi Jia Cang Fang Jie

YANG YIN GAO

Main Ingredients

Sha Shen (Radix adenophorae strictae)	250 grams
Yu Zhu (Rhizoma polygonati odorati)	250 grams
Mai Dong (Radix ophopogonis)	250 grams
Hua Fen (Pollen)	250 grams
Bai He (Bulbus lilii)	250 grams

Preparation

Decoct the above ingredients. Condense the decoction and add an adequate amount of refined honey.

Dosage and Administration

Take 2–3 times daily, 15 grams each time.

Effect

Nourishes *yin*, promotes the production of body fluids, moistens and strengthens the lungs and stomach, and calms the mind to relieve restlessness.

Indications

Dry mouth and throat, dry cough with scanty expectoration, restlessness, palpitations (all due to over consumption of body fluids caused by *yin* deficiency of the lung and stomach).

2.4.4 SOFT EXTRACT FOR SUPPORTING *YANG*

SUO YANG GAO

Main Ingredients

Suo Yang (Herba cynoniorii)	1500 grams

Preparation

Suo Yang is decocted in water, the decoction is then condensed. Mix the condensed decoction evenly with 250 grams of refined honey.

Dosage and Administration

Take orally, twice daily, 30 grams each time.

Effect

Reinforces the kidney-*yang*, supplements the essence and blood, and moistens the intestines.

Indications

Insufficiency of kidney-*yang*, consumption and deficiency of the vital essence and blood, and constipation due to over consumption of body fluids caused by dryness in the intestines.

Source

Ben Cao Qie Yao

CONG RONG ER XIAN GAO

Main Ingredients

Rou Cong Rong (Herba cistanchis)	500 grams
Yin Yang Huo (Herba epirnedii)	500 grams
Xian Mao (Rhizoma curculiginis)	250 grams

Preparation

Decoct the above ingredients. Condense the decoction and add an adequate amount of refined honey.

Dosage and Administration

Take orally, twice daily in the morning and evening, 15 grams each time.

Effect

Reinforces the kidney-*yang*, strengthens tendons and bones, and eliminates cold-dampness.

Indications

Insufficiency of the kidney-*yang,* impotence; weakness of the loins and knees; flaccidity of the extremities; and disorders due to wind, cold, and dampness; and numbness of the limbs.

Notes

Because of its dry and heat-nature, patients that do not have syndrome due to *Yang* deficiency should not take this medicine regularly.

Main Ingredients
Ge Jie (Gecko)
Dang Shen (Radix codonopsis)
Dosage Form
Soft extract, 250 grams in each bottle.
Dosage and Administration
Take with warm boiled water, twice daily, 10 grams each time.
Effect
Invigorates the kidneys, supports *yang*, tonifies the lungs,
strengthens the spleen, relieves cough, and arrests asthma.
Indications
Chronic cough, anemia, sallow complexion, and indigestion
due to deficiency of the kidney-*yang* and the lung-*yin*.
Manufacturer
Nanjing Pharmaceutical Factory of Traditional Chinese
Medicines in Guangxi

2.4.5 SOFT EXTRACT FOR TONIFYING BOTH *QI* AND BLOOD

Main Ingredients

Ren Shen (Radix ginseng)	120 grams
Shu Di (Rhiaoma rehmanniae praeparata)	500 grams

Preparation
Decoct the above ingredients. Condense the decoction and
add an adequate amount of refined honey.
Dosage and Administration
Take orally, twice daily in the morning and evening, 15 grams
each time.
Effect
Invigorates the primordial *qi*, and nourishes *yin*-blood.
Indications
Insufficiency of vital essence and *qi* in the interior and
deficiency of *yin*-blood.
Source
Jing Yue Quan Shu
Notes
This is a mild extract for tonifing *qi* and blood. It may be taken
regularly. *Ren Shen* may be replaced with 250 grams of *Dang
Shen (Radix codonopsis pilosulae)*.

Main Ingredients

Dang Shen (Radix codonopsis)	500 grams
Mi Zhi Huang Qi (honeyed *Radix astragali*)	500 grams
Chao Bai Zhu (parched *Rhizoma atractylodis macrocephalae*)	500 grams

Chao Bai Shao (parched *Radix paeoniae alba*)	500 grams
Fu Ling (Poria)	500 grams
Shu Di Huang (Rhizoma rehmanniae praeparata)	750 grams
Dang Gui (Radix angelicae sinensis)	750 grams
Chuan Xiong (Rhizoma chuanxiong)	250 grams
Rou Gui (Cortex cinnamomi)	250 grams
Mi Zhi Gan Cao (Radix glycyrrhizae praeparata)	250 grams

Preparation

Decoct the above ingredients in water. Condense the decoction. Dissolve 530 grams of granulated sugar in water, heat it and filter it. Mix the sugar with 1000 grams of the condensed decoction into a soft extract.

Dosage and Administration

Dissolve the soft extract in boiling water and take before a meal, twice daily, 15 grams each time.

Effect

Warms and tonifies the primordial *qi*.

Indications

Syndromes due to deficiency of *qi* and blood.

Source

Jiang Su Sheng Yao Pin Biao Zhun

YANG SHEN SHUANG BU GAO

Main Ingredients

Xi Yang Shen (Radix panacis quinquefolii)	30 grams
Shan Yao (Rhizoma dioscoreae)	500 grams
Gou Qi Zi (Fructus lycii)	500 grams
Sang Shen Zi (Fructus niori)	750 grams
Da Zao (Fructus jujubae)	750 grams
Long Yao Rou (Arillus longan)	750 grams

Preparation

Decoct the above ingredients. Condense the decoction and add an adequate amount of refined honey.

Dosage and Administration

Take orally, twice daily, 30 grams each time.

Effect

Nourishes the blood, enriches *yin*, and mildly tonifies the heart, spleen, liver and kidney.

Indications

Syndromes due to deficiency of *qi* and insufficiency of blood and consumption of *yin*.

Notes

All the herbs except *Xi Yang Shen* are edible. As *Xi Yang Shen* is rare and expensive, it may be replaced with *Tai Zi Shen* (Radix pseudostellariae) in a dosage of ten times that of *Xi Yang Shen*.

2.4.6 SOFT EXTRACTS FOR TONIFYING THE FIVE *ZANG* ORGANS

GOU QI GAO

Main Ingredients

Gou Qi Zi (Fructus lycii)	500 grams

Preparation
Decoct the above ingredients. Condense the decoction and add an adequate amount of refined honey.

Dosage and Administration
Take orally, twice daily in the morning and evening, 15–30 grams each time.

Effect
Tonifies the liver and kidneys, nourishes *yin*, moistens the lungs, and improves eyesight.

Indications
Disorders due to *yin* deficiency of the liver and kidneys, such as dizziness, blurring of vision, soreness and weakness of the loins and knees, and cough.

Source
Shou Shi Bao Yuan

CANG ZHU GAO

Main Ingredients

Cang Zhu (Rhizoma atractylodis)	500 grams
Fu Ling (Poria)	500 grams

Preparation
Decoct the above ingredients. Condense the decoction and add an adequate amount of refined honey or granulated sugar.

Dosage and Administration
Take orally, 2–3 times daily, 15–30 grams each time.

Effect
Strengthens the spleen and stomach and replenishes *qi*.

Indications
Poor appetite, decline of vigor, amnesia, insomnia, and edema, soreness and heavy feeling of the legs and feet, and weakness of the spleen and stomach.

Source
Wei Sheng Za Xing Fang

FU LING GAO

Main Ingredients

Fu Ling (Poria)	1000 grams
Song Zhi (Colophonium)	500 grams
Song Zi Ren (Semen pini)	250 grams
Bai Zi Ren (Semen biotae)	250 grams

Preparation
Steam and dry *Fu Ling* seven times. Grind all the ingredients

into a powder, sift it, and mix it with 1000 grams of honey. Place the mixture into a bronze container with water and decoct it over a mild heat for a day and night into a soft extract.

Dosage and Administration

Take three times daily, 15–30 grams each time.

Effect

Nourishes the heart, calms the mind, and strengthens the body.

Indications

Disturbed mind, palpitations, insomnia, and amnesia.

Source

Tai Ping Sheng Hui Fang

RUN FEI GAO

Main Ingredients

Nan Sha Shen (Radix adenophorae)	50 grams
Mai Dong (Radix ophiopogonis)	50 grams
Tian Dong (Radix asparagi)	50 grams
Hua Fen (Pollen)	50 grams
Pi Pa Ye (Folium eriobotryae)	50 grams
Xing Ren (Semen armeniacae amarum)	50 grams
He Tao Ren (Sernen juglandis)	50 grams
Bing Tang (crystal sugar)	50 grams
Chuan Bei Mu (Bulbus fritillariae cirrhosae)	120 grams
Ju Bing (orange in the form of cake)	250 grams

Preparation

Remove the hair of *Pi Pa Ye* and grind *Chuan Bei Mu* and *Bing Tang* into separate powders. Decoct the ingredients except Chuan, *Bei Mu* and *Bing Tang* in water and concentrate the decoction. Mix the thick decoction with the powder of *Chuan Bei Mu* and *Bing Tang* and 6000 grams of honey into soft extract.

Dosage and Administration

Take orally, twice daily, 15 grams each time.

Effect

Nourishes the lung-*yin*, relieves cough, and reduces phlegm.

Indications

Disorders due to dryness in the lung caused by *yin* deficiency, such as dry mouth and throat, unproductive cough, and cough with little but sticky sputum.

Source

Jiang Su Sheng Yao Pin Biao Zhun

2.4.7 OTHER SOFT EXTRACTS FOR TONIFYING THE BODY AND PROLONGING LIFE

QIONG YÜ GAO

Main Ingredients

Ren Shen (Radix ginseng)	75 grams
Sheng Di (Radix rehmanniae)	800 grams
Fu Ling (Poria)	153 grams
Bai Mi (Mel)	500 grams

Preparation
Refine *Bai Mi*, grind the other ingredients into a powder, and decoct in water. Condense the decoction and mixed with the refined honey into soft extract.

Dosage and Administration
Take orally, 2–3 times daily, 15 grams each time.

Effect
Invigorates *qi* and *yin*, promotes the production of vital essence and blood, nourishes the kidneys, enhances the lungs, strengthens the spleen and stomach, and tonifies the heart.

Indications
Unproductive cough due to deficiency and consumption, dry throat, and hemoptysis.

Source
Hong Shi Ji Yan Fang compiled by Hong Zun in the Song dynasty.

Notes
The dosage and ingredients have been modified according to the original prescription in the book. For example, ingredients as such *Chen Xiang (Lignurn aquilariae resinatum)* and *Hu Po (Succinurn)* are sometimes added. This extract will help restore *qi*, strengthen the body's resistance, consolidate the constitution, expel phlegm, and slow down the process of aging.

Recent research has shown that this extract can increase the count of T-lymphocytes and reducing the content of serum IgA in the old.

YI SHOU YANG ZHEN GAO

Main Ingredients

Sheng Di Huang (Rhizoma rehmanniae praeparata)	8000 grams
Ren Shen (Radix ginseng)	750 grams
Fu Ling (Poria)	1500 grams
Mi (Mel)	5000 grams
Tian Dong (Radix asparagi)	250 grams
Mai Dong (Radix ophiopogonis)	250 grams
Di Gu Pi (Cortex lycii)	250 grams

Preparation

Grind all of the above ingredients except *Mi* into a powder. Mix in *Mi* thoroughly and place in a porcelain jar. Seal the jar, place it in a bronze pot, and boil in water for 72 hours. Keep adding warm water to the boiling pot so that it does not dry out. When the boiling is complete, seal the jar with wax paper and place it in a dark place for 24 hours. Finally, place the jar in the pot again and boil it for another 24 hours.

Dosage and Administration

Take after being mixed with warm liquor, 2–3 times daily, 1–2 teaspoons each time.

Effect and **Indications**

The same as those of *Qiong Yü Gao*

HE CHE GAO

Main Ingredients

Dang Shen (Radix codonopsis)	60 grams
Sheng Di (Radix rehmanniae)	60 grams
Gou Qi Zi (Fructus lycii)	60 grams
Dang Gui (Radix angelicae sinensis)	60 grams
Zi He Che (Placenta hominis)	one

Preparation

Decoct the above ingredients. Condense the decoction and add an adequate amount of refined honey or granulated sugar.

Dosage and Administration

Take in the morning, after being mixed with millet wine, 3–5 spoons each time.

Effect

Enriches *qi*, nourishes the blood, supports *yang*, replenishes *yin*, supplements marrow, and tonifies the liver and kidneys.

Indications

General debility and insufficiency of *qi*, blood, and *yin* and *yang*.

Source

It has another name, *Hun Yuan Gao*, and is recorded the book, *Qing Tai Yi Yuan Pei Fang*.

Notes

This extract can be used to treat men and women with syndromes due to various kinds of deficiencies and injuries, such as:

• the five kinds of strains and the seven kinds of impairments
• susceptibility to diseases and intolerance of strain due to weakness of the primordial qi from congenital factors
• impotence and sterility due to deficiency of the kidney
• frequent miscarriage due to cold of the deficiency type in the uterus.

GUI LU ER XIAN GAO

Main Ingredients

Lu Jiao (Cornu cervi)	500 grams
Gui Ban (Carapax et plastrum testudinis)	250 grams
Gou Qi Zi (Fructus lycii)	100 grams
Ren Shen (Radix ginseng)	50 grams

Preparation

Cut up *Lu Jiao* and *Gui Ban* and scrape them clean. Steep them in water and decoct over a mulberry-leaf fire into a gum. Decoct *Gou Qi Zi* and *Ren Shen* in water. Mix the decoction with the gum into a soft extract.

Dosage and Administration

Take in the morning, after being mixed with wine, 9 grams each time.

Effect

Warms *yang*, benefits *yin*, nourishes the liver and kidneys, and invigorates *qi*, blood, essence and marrow.

Indications

Consumptive diseases, exhaustion of essence, nocturnal emissions, emaciation, languor, and blurred vision.

Source

Xian Chuan Si Shi Jiu Fang.

HONG YU GAO

Main Ingredients

Yu Zhu (Rhizoma polygonati odorati)	90 grams
Ren Shen (Radix ginseng)	90 grams
Wu Wei Zi (Fructus schisandrae)	60 grams
Gui Ban Jiao (Colla carapacis et Plastri testudinis)	60 grams
Dang Gui (Radix Angelicae sinensis)	60 grams
Da Sheng Di (Radix rebrnanniac)	60 grams
Fu Ling (Poria)	60 grams
Gou Qi Zi (Fructus lycli)	60 grams
Chuan Niu Xi (Radix achyranthis bidentatae)	30 grams
Bai Lian Xu (Stamen nelumbinis)	15 grams
Zhu Sha (Cinnabaris)	3 grams

Preparation

Decoct the above ingredients. Condense the decoction and add an adequate amount of refined honey or granulated sugar.

Dosage and Administration

Take orally, 2–3 times daily, 15 grams each time.

Effect

Supplements the vital essence and marrow, consolidates *qi*, nourishes the blood, regulates the five *Zang* organs, enhances the nine orifices, and greatly benefits health.

Indications

Senility due to deficiency and impairments.

Source

Ji Yan Liang Fang in the Qing dynasty

Main Ingredients

Dang Shen (Radix codonopsis)	45 grams
Bai Zhu (Rhizoma atractylodis macrocephalae baked in earth)	30 grams
Fu Ling (Poria)	30 grams
Dang Gui (Radix angelicae sinensis baked in earth)	30 grams
Xu Duan (Radix dipsaci parched with liquor)	30 grams
Huang Qi (Radix astragah)	30 grams
Chao Gu Ya (parched Fructus oryzae germinatus)	30 grams
Ji Nei Jin (Endothelium corneum gigeriae galli roasted)	30 grams
Zhi Ban Xia (Rhizoma pinelliae praeparata)	24 grams
Sheng Jiang (Rhizoma zingiberis)	24 grams
Zhi Xiang Fu (Rhizoma cyperi praeparata)	18 grams
Shu Di (Rhizoma rehmanniae praeparata)	18 grams
Sha Ren (Fructus amomi)	12 grams
Pei Lan Cao (Herba eupatorii)	12 grams
Hong Zao Rou (Fructus jujubae with the core removed)	20 dates

Preparation

Decoct the above ingredients. Condense the decoction and add an adequate amount of refined honey or granulated sugar.

Dosage and Administration

Take with boiled water, 9 grams each time.

Effect

Strengthens the spleen, replenishes qi, nourishes the blood, promotes digestion to eliminate retained food, and tonifies the liver and kidneys.

Indications

General debility due to prolonged illness, weakness of the spleen and stomach, poor appetite, distension in the abdomen, retching, hiccups, and indigestion.

Source

Ci Xi Guang Yu Yi Fang Xuan Yi

Notes

This prescription was established especially for the sake of Cixi Empress Dowager during the Qing dynasty.

Main Ingredients

Dang Shen (Radix codonopsis)	60 grams
Chao Bai Zhu (parched Rhizoma atractylodis macrocephalae)	30 grams
Fu Ling (Poria)	30 grams
Shan Yao (Rhizoma dioscoreae)	30 grams
Dang Gui (Radix angelicae sinensis baked in earth)	30 grams

Nü Zhen Zi (Fructus ligustri lucidi)	30 grams
Bai Shao (Radix paeoniae alba parched with vinegar)	24 grams
Dan Pi (Cortex moutan)	18 grams
Zhi Xiang Fu (Rhizoma cyperi praeparata)	18 grams
Lu Jiao Jiao (Colla cornus cervi melted)	15 grams
Sha Ren (Fructus arnomi)	12 grams
Yin Chai Hu (Radix stellariae)	9 grams

Preparation

Decoct all of the above ingredients except *Lu Jiao Jiao* in water thoroughly. Concentrate the decoction and mix evenly with the melted *Lu Jiao Jiao,* and add an adequate amount of refined honey into soft extract.

Dosage and Administration

Take with boiled water, 12 grams each time.

Effect

This prescription is a modification of *Xiao Yao San.* It strengthens the spleen, replenishes *qi,* regulates the liver and spleen to promote the flow of *qi,* warms the kidneys, invigorates *yin,* and nourishes the blood.

Indications

Consumptive diseases due to stagnation of the liver *qi*

Source

Ci Xi Guang Xu Yi Fang Xuan Yi

2.4.8 SOFT EXTRACTS FOR HEALTHCARE USED TO PREVENT AND TREAT DISEASES

JU HUA YAN LING GAO

Main Ingredients

Xian Ju Hua (*Flos chrysanthemi*), fresh and in an adequate amount

Preparation

Decoct *Xian Ju Hua* in water thoroughly. Concentrate the decoction and mix it with small amount of refined honey into a soft extract.

Dosage and Administration

Take with boiled water, 9–12 grams each time.

Effect

Dispels wind, clears away heat, calms the liver, and improves eyesight.

Indications

Dizziness, blurred vision, headache and conjunctival congestion due to hyperfunction of the liver *yang* and wind-heat pathogens.

Source

Ci Xi Guang Xu Yi Fang Xuan Yi

Notes

This prescription was established specially for Cixi Empress Dowager. Modern pharmacological and clinical studies discovered that this extract may be used to treat hypertension and coronary heart disease.

Main Ingredients

Shuang Sang Ye (Folium mori)	30 grams
Ju Hua (Flos chrysanthemi)	30 grams

Preparation

Decoct the above ingredients. Condense the decoction and add an adequate amount of refined honey or granulated sugar.

Dosage and Administration

Take with boiled water, 9 grams each time.

Effect and Indications

Similar to those of *Ju Hua Yan Ling Gao*

Source

Ci Xi Guang Xu Yi Fang Xuan Yi

Main Ingredients

Huang Li (pear)	100 pears
Xian Zhu Ye (fresh Herba Lophatheri)	100 pieces
Xian Lu Gen (fresh Rhizoma Phragmitis)	30 pieces
Lao Shu Ju Hong (Exocarpiumcitri grandis)	20 pieces
Bi Qi (bulbus Eleocharis tuberosae)	50 pieces
Zhu Li (Succus barnbusae)	adequate amount

Preparation

Decoct the above ingredients. Condense the decoction and add an adequate amount of refined honey or granulated sugar.

Effect

Nourishes yin to promote the production of body fluids, moistens the lungs to arrest cough, and clears away heat to eliminate phlegm.

Indications

Dryness in the lungs caused by yin deficiency

Source

Ci Xi Guang Xu Yi Fang Xuan Yi

Main Ingredients

Mai Dong (Radix ophiopogonis)	100 grams
Pang Da Hai (Semen sterculiae lychnophorae)	100 grams
Tian Hua Fen (Radix trichosanthis)	100 grams
Huang Li (pear)	1000 grams
Xian Qing Guo (fresh *Fructus canarii*)	500 grams
Jie Geng (Radix platycodi)	50 grams
Mu Hu Die (Semen oroxyli)	50 grams
Gan Cao (Radix glycyrrhizae)	30 grams

| Shuang Hua (Flos lonicerae) | 75 grams |
| Shi Shuang (Mannosum kaki) | 30 grams |

Preparation

Decoct all of the above ingredients in water except *Shi Shuang*. Condense the decoction, mix with *Shi Shuang*, and add an adequate amount of refined honey into a soft extract.

Dosage and Administration

Take with boiled water or orally, three times daily, 9–15 grams each time.

Effect

Clears away heat, replenishes *yin*, promotes the production of body fluids, and relieves sore throats.

Indications

Sore throat, dry mouth and throat, and hoarseness.

SHOU WU JU ZHA GAO

Main Ingredients

He Shou Wu (Radix polygoni multiflori)	500 grams
Ju Hua (Flos chrysanthemi)	500 grams
Sheng Shan Zha (Fructus crataegi)	500 grams

Preparation

Decoct the above ingredients. Condense the decoction and add an adequate amount of refined honey or granulated sugar.

Dosage and Administration

Take three times daily, 10–15 grams each time.

Effect

Nourishes the liver and kidneys, calms the liver to improve eyesight, and activates blood circulation.

Indications

Hypertension, hyperlipernia, and coronary heart disease.

YI QI HUO XUE GAO

Main Ingredients

Huang Qi (Radix astragali)	500 grams
Dan Shen (Radix salviae miltiorrhizae)	500 grams
Huang Jing (Rhizoma polygonati)	250 grams
Yu Jin (Radix curcurnae)	250 grams
Sheng Shan Zha (Fructus crataegi)	250 grams

Preparation

Decoct the above ingredients. Condense the decoction and add an adequate amount of refined honey or granulated sugar.

Dosage and Administration

Take three times daily, 15 grams each time.

Effect

Replenishes *qi* and promotes the circulation of blood.

Indications

Indications include all the disorders due to deficiency of *qi* and stagnation of blood, such as coronary heart disease, chronic

obstructive pulmonary emphysema, and chronic pulmonary
heart disease in the remission stage.

LAO GUAN CAO GAO

Main Ingredients

Lao Guan Cao (Herba erodiiseu geranii)	500 grams
Dang Gui (Radix Angelicae sinensis)	125 grams
Bai Xian Pi (Cortex dictarnni)	62.5 grams
Chuan Xiong (Rhizoma chuanxiong)	62.5 grams
Hong Hua (Flos cartharni)	31 grams

Preparation

Decoct the above ingredients. Condense the decoction and
add an adequate amount of refined honey or granulated sugar.

Dosage and Administration

Take 2-3 times, 9-15 grams each time.

Effect

Expels wind-dampness and promotes blood circulation to
remove obstruction in the channels.

Indications

Pain due to pathogenic wind-dampness, stiff muscles and
tendons, spasm and numbness of the limbs, traumatic injury,
and itchy skin.

Source

Qing Tai Yi Yuan Pei Fang

2.5 Chinese Herbal Tea for Healthcare

Chinese herbal teas are of two types. One, known as *Dai Cha Yin*, is
a coarse powder with or without tea leaves. It is steeped in boiling
water and then taken orally. *Dai Cha Yin* aids in the maintaining of
one's health. The other type of herbal tea, *Wu Shi Cha*, exists in the
form of lumps of coarse powder mixed with flour paste or medicated
leaven. It is also steeped in boiling water and then taken orally. *Wu Shi
Cha* is produced by pharmaceutical factories and is not discussed in this
section.

China is the home of tea and has seen several thousand years of
cultivating and drinking it. Tea is a fine beverage that can relieve thirst
and restlessness, resolve phlegm, promote digestion, induce diuresis,
eliminate toxic substances, and refresh oneself. Thus tea has long
enjoyed popularity in China.

It was found in Chinese history that tea could be mixed with
suitable medicines to prevent and treat diseases and that some medicines might be substituted for tea and infused with boiling water for
oral use. Hence, *Dai Cha Yin* (herbal tea used to prevent and treat
diseases or to maintain one's health and prolong life) came into being.

Herbal teas have many unique merits, such as:
- They are in small doses.
- They save drug material.
- They can be taken just after being infused with boiling water without the need to be decocted over fire.
- They are easier to prepare and more suitable for long-standing administration than decoctions.
- They can be prescribed either for drug therapy, dietetic therapy, or prevention and treatment of disease.
- They can be enjoyed by the old and the young.

Dai Cha Yin is a widely used herbal tea type. It is used for the treatment of mild cases, chronic diseases, and serious diseases, for the protection of health, and for the retardation of senility. Additionally, regular intake of *Dai Cha Yin* will help prevent and treat disorders in the oral cavity, throat, esophagus, stomach, and intestines.

Dai Cha Yin is characterized by its medicine, administration, prescription, and composition. Medicines administered in it are usually mild-natured, sweet and mild tasting—such as fruits, vegetables, sugar, and honey—which are edible and easy to obtain. The ingredients of a prescription of *Dai Cha Yin* usually number between 5–7; the amount of each ingredient is generally not over 10 grams , and the dose of a whole prescription is small. In spite of the above characteristic, a *Dai Cha Yin's* composition and the compatibility of its ingredients are both strictly based on overall analysis and differentiation of all the factors concerned.

The preparation of *Dai Cha Yin* is simple. Select high-quality and clean herbs and remove any dust and impurities in them if necessary. Break up the herbs into coarse powder. Be sure that it is not too fine because it will make the tea turbid. Place the powder into filter pouches so that one pouch may be administered each time. Be sure to keep the powder and pouches dry.

When preparing *Dai Cha Yin* steep the pouch in boiling water as if you were making tea and drink.

Dai Cha Yin should be prescribed according to the differentiation of an individual's constitution, disease state, and age as well as the particular season in order to achieve the best results. It is important to remember that *Dai Cha Yin*, because it is taken in small doses and is mild in nature, should not be the sole treatment for emergency and severe cases lest the opportunity to cure them be missed. When *Dai Cha Yin* is used for healthcare and longevity, the effects will be ensured only by its long-term, regular administration.

The following are various kinds of herbal teas used for healthcare.

2.5.1 HERBAL TEA FOR INVIGORATING *QI* AND ENRICHING BLOOD

SHEN QI DAI CHA YIN

Main Ingredients

Ren Shen (Radix ginseng)	3 grams
Huang Qi (Radix astragali)	9 grams
Da Zao (Fructus jujubae)	5 dates
Chen Pi (Pericarpium citri reticulatae)	1.5 grams

Preparation and Administration

Infuse the above ingredients with boiling water and take as tea.

Effect

Invigorates primordial *qi* without causing any stagnation, strengthens the spleen and stomach, and delays senility.

Indications

Regular in take of this tea is suitable for those who are weak due to the deficiency of *qi*.

Notes

Ren Shen may be substituted by *Dang Shen* (*Radix codonopsis*).

WU BAO CHA TANG

Main Ingredients

Shu Mi Mian (broomcom millet flour)
Zhi Ma (*Semen sesanii*)
Niu Ru (milk)
Shan Yao (*Rhizoma dioscoreae*)
Niu Gu Sui (ox marrow)

Preparation and Administration

Grind *Zhi Ma* and *Shan Yao* into a powder. Dissolve *Niu Gu Sui* in sesame oil. Parch *Shu Mi Mian*. Mix the above processed ingredients evenly with *Niu Ru* and *Wu Bao Cha Tang*. Infuse with boiling water and take every morning.

Effect

Invigorates *qi*, strengthens the spleen, replenishes vital essence, enriches the blood, and nourishes the liver and kidneys.

Indications

Taking this regularly is included in dietetic therapy.

Source

Ren Shou Lu

GUAN YIN MIAN CHA

Main Ingredients

Chao Hei Zhi Ma (parched *Semen sesami*)	500 grams
Ou Fen (lotus root starch)	500 grams
Nian Huang Mi (glutinous yellow rice)	500 grams
Bai Tang (white sugar)	500 grams
Chao Shan Yao (parched *Rhizoma dioscoreae*)	500 grams

Preparation and Administration

Grind the above ingredients into a fine powder. Infuse an appropriate amount with boiling water for oral use.

Effect

Replenishes *qi*, strengthens the spleen, invigorates vital essence, enriches the blood, and nourishes the liver and kidney.

Indications

Suitable for those weak and senile.

Source

Ren Shou Lu

WU XIANG NAI CHA

Main Ingredients

Niu Ru (milk)
Bai Sha Tang (white granulated sugar)
Feng Mi (Mel)
Xing Ren (Semen armeniacae amarum)
Zhi Ma (Semen sesame)

Preparation and Administration

Break *Xing Ren* and *Zhi Ma* into coarse powder and mix evenly with *Bai Sha Tang* and *Feng Mi*. Heat *Niu Ru* and pour into the mixture.

Effect

Replenishes *qi*, supplements vital essence, enriches the blood, moistens the lungs, relaxes the bowels, and nourishes the liver and kidneys.

Indications

This tea is especially applicable to those who are infirm with age and have the symptoms of cough and constipation.

Source

Ren Shou Lu

ZHU DONG DAI CHA YIN

Main Ingredients

Bai Zhu (Rhizoma atractylodis macrocephalae)	4.5 grams
Mai Dong (Radix ophiopogonis with pith removed)	3 grams

Preparation and Administration

Infuse the above ingredients in water during the summer and taken as tea.

Effect

Invigorates *qi*, strengthens the spleen, nourishes *yin*, and moistens the heart and lungs.

Indications

It is suitable for those with syndromes due to deficiency of the spleen-*qi* or *yin* deficiency of the heart and lung.

Source

Chuan Ya Nei Wai Pian

SANG LONG DAI CHA YIN

Main Ingredients

Sang Shen Zi (Fructus mori)	15 grams
Long Yan Rou (Arillus longan)	15 grams

Preparation and Administration

Infuse the above ingredients in boiling water and drink as tea.

Effect

This herbal tea acts mainly in enriching the blood. It also replenishes *yin*, invigorates *qi*, nourishes the heart, tranquilizes the mind, promotes the production of body fluids, and moistens the intestines.

Indications

Deficiency of the vital essence and blood, dizziness, tinnitus, insomnia, amnesia, severe palpitation, anorexia, weariness, early graying of hair, and constipation due to dry feces.

YI QI SHENG JIN DAI CHA YIN

Main Ingredients

Ren Shen (Radix ginseng)
Xian Shi Hu (fresh *Herba dendrobli*)
Mai Dong (Radix ophiopogonis)
Xian Qing Guo (fresh *Fructus canarii*)
Lao Mi (long-stored rice)

Effect

Replenishes *qi*, nourishes *yin*, promotes the production of body fluids, removes heat, and relieves sore throats.

Indications

Deficiency of *qi* and *yin*, consumption and lack of body fluids, dry mouth, and dry and sore throats.

BU XUE HE WEI DAI CHA YIN

Main Ingredients

Dang Gui Shen (*Radix angelicae sinensis,* middle part is used)
Chuan Xiong (Rhizoma chuanxiong)
Bai Shao (Radix paeoniae alba)
Sheng Di (Radix relunanniae)
Guang Mu Xiang (Radix saussureae lappae)
Zhi Shi (Fructus Aurantii immaturus)

Cang Zhu (Rhizoma atractylodis)
Jiao San Xian (parched *Massa fermentata medicinalis*)
Fructus crataegi parched
Fructus hordei germinatus parched
Effect
Enriches the blood
Indications
Dysfunction of the spleen and stomach and deficiency of *yin*-blood.

2.5.2 HERBAL TEA FOR NOURISHING *YIN* AND SUPPORTING *YANG*

YU SHI DAI CHA YIN

Main Ingredients

Yu Zhu (Rhizoma polygonati odorati)	6 grams
Shi Hu (Herba dendrobil)	6 grams

Preparation and Administration
Infuse the above ingredients in boiling water and drink as tea.
Effect
Nourishes *yin*, moistens dryness, and promotes the production of body fluid.
Indications
Syndrome due to *yin* deficiency of the lungs and stomach indicated by dry and heat cough, dry mouth and tongue due to the consumption of body fluid, weakness and soreness of the loins and knees, blurred vision, and diabetes.

ER SHEN ER DONG DAI CHA YIN

Main Ingredients

Sha Shen (Radix adenophorae)	6 grams
Xuan Shen (Radix scrophulariae)	6 grams
Mai Dong (Radix ophiopogonis)	6 grams
Tian Dong (Radix asparagi)	6 grams

Effect
Nourishes *yin*, promotes the production of body fluids, and clears away heat.
Indications
Yin impairment of the lung and stomach indicated by dry mouth and throat, dry cough with little sputum, and anorexia. *Yin* impairment due to febrile disease indicated by restlessness, insomnia, flaring-up of fire of the deficiency type, congestion of the eye(s), sore throat, and constipation caused by dry feces.
Notes
Those with constitution of *yin*-deficiency type can take the above two herbal teas.

SHEN LING DAI CHA YIN

Main Ingredients

Sha Shen (Radix adenophorae)
Fu Ling (Poria)
Tian Dong (Radix asparagi)

Effect

Nourishes *yin* and supports the spleen.

Indications

Syndrome due to *yin* deficiency of the lung, stomach, and kidneys and complicated by the deficiency of the spleen.

XIAN LING PI CHA

Main Ingredients

Yin Yang Huo (Herba epiniedii)	9 grams
Rou Cong Rong (Herba cistanchis)	6 grams

Preparation and Administration

Infuse the above ingredients in boiling water and drink as tea.

Effect

Supplements kidney-*yang*, strengthens the tendons and bones, and replenishes the vital essence and blood.

Indications

Impotence, infertility, weakness of the loins and knees, cold pain, hypertension, and coronary heart disease (all due to deficiency of the kidney-*yang*).

FU FANG DU ZHONG CHA

Main Ingredients

Du Zhong (Cortex eucommiae)	9 grams
Sang Ji Sheng (Ramulus taxilliseu visci)	9 grams
Huai Niu Xi (Radix achyranthis bidentatae)	9 grams

Preparation and Administration

Infuse the above ingredients in boiling water and drink as tea.

Effect

Tonifies the liver and kidneys and strengthens tendons and bones.

Indications

Lumbago and weakness of the feet and knees due to deficiency of the kidney and hypertension with symptoms due to deficiency of the liver and kidney.

XIN ER XIAN DAI CHA YIN

Main Ingredients

Xian Mao (Rhizoma curculiginis)	4.5 grams
Yin Yang Huo (Herba epimedii)	6 grams
Du Zhong (Cortex eucommiae)	6 grams

Xuan Shen (Radix scrophulariae)	6 grams
Nü Zhen Zi (Fructrus ligustri lucidi)	6 grams
Gou Qi Zi (Fructus lycii)	6 grams

Preparation and Administration

Infuse the above ingredients in boiling water and drink as tea.

Effect

Tonifies the liver and kidneys, warms *yang*, nourishes *yin*, and removes fire.

Indications

Syndrome due to deficiency of *yin* and *yang* in both the liver and kidneys and hypertension and coronary heart disease with symptoms due to the above syndrome.

FU FANG GOU QI CHA

Main Ingredients

Gou Qi Zi (Fructus lycii)	6 grams
Bai He (Bulbus lilii)	6 grams
He Shou Wu (Radix polygoni multiflori)	6 grams
Huang Jing (Rhizoma polygonati)	6 grams
Yin Yang Huo (Herba epimedii)	6 grams

Preparation and Administration

Infuse the above ingredients in boiling water and drink as tea.

Effect

Mildly reinforces *qi*, blood, and *yin* and *yang* with the five *zang* organs. Aids in retarding senility, building up the constitution, and prolonging life.

Indications

This tea is suitable for those that are weak, middle-aged or elderly.

2.5.3 HERBAL TEA FOR REGULATING THE FUNCTION OF THE SPLEEN AND STOMACH TO PROMOTE DIGESTION

HE WEI DAI CHA YIN

Main Ingredients

Sheng Bai Zhu (Rhizoma atractylodis macrocephalae)
Cang Zhu (Rhizoma atractylodis)
Fu Ling (Poria)
Chen Pi (Pericarpium citri reticulatae)
Jin Shi Hu (Herba dendrobii)
Gu Ya (Fructus oryzae germinatus)
Jian Qu (Massa medicata fermentata)
Guang Sha Ren (Fructus amomi)

Effect

Strengthens the spleen and stomach, nourishes *yin,* and promotes digestion.

Indications

Syndrome due to weakness of the spleen and stomach end complicated by *yin* deficiency of the stomach and indicated by anorexia and food retention.

Source

Qing Dai Gong Ting Yi Hua

Notes

It is recorded in the book, *Qing Dai Gong Ting Yi Hua*, that this prescription was one of those for regulation and invigoration once used to treat the emperor *Guang Xu* after his illness.

ER SHEN DAI CHA YIN

Main Ingredients

Fu Shen (Poria cum ligno hospite)

Shen Qu (Massa fermentata medicinalis)

Effect

Strengthens the spleen, calms the mind, and regulates the stomach to promote digestion.

Indications

Deficiency of the spleen, anorexia, indigestion, and uneasiness.

Wu Xian Dai Cha Yin

Main Ingredients

Shen Qu (Massa fermentata medicinalis)	6 grams
Chao Shan Zha (parched *Fructus crataegi*)	6 grams
Chao Mai Ya (parched *Fructus hordei germinatus*)	6 grams
Chao Gu Ya (parched *Fructus oryzae germinatus*)	6 grams
Sha Ren (Fructus arnorni)	3 grams

Preparation and Administration

Infuse the above ingredients in boiling water and drink as tea.

Effect

Promotes digestion and removes any stagnation and food retention. It also activates the flow of *qi* and regulates the function of the stomach.

Indications

Food retention, distention and fullness in the stomach and abdomen, and belching with disagreeable odors of undigested food.

GAN LU CHA

Main Ingredients

Wu Yao (Radix linderae)	24 grams
Chao Hou Po (parched *Cortex magnoliae officinalis*)	24 grams
Chao Zhi Shi (parched *Fructus aurantii*)	24 grams
Chao Shan Zha (parched *Fructus crataegi*)	24 grams
Chen Pi (Pericarpium citri reticulatae)	120 grams
Chao Shen Qu (parched *Massa fermentata medicinalis*)	45 grams
Chao Gu Ya (parched *Fructus oryzae germinatus*)	30 grams
Hong Cha (black tea)	90 grams

Preparation

Grind the above ingredients into coarse powder and mix evenly. Place 9 grams of the powder into pouches.

Administration

One pouch and one piece of *Sheng Jiang* (Rhizoma zingiberis recens) are decocted or steeped in boiling water for oral use.

Effect

Regulates the flow of *qi*, promotes digestion, and removes stagnation.

Indications

Food retention, *qi* stagnation, distending and depressing sensation in the stomach and abdomen, and anorexia.

Source

Yao Ji Xue

2.5.4 HERBAL TEA FOR TRANQUILIZING THE MIND

AN SHEN DAI CHA YIN

Main Ingredients

Duan Long Chi (forged *Os draconis*)	9 grams
Shi Chang Pu (Rhizoma acori graminei)	3 grams

Preparation and Administration

Infuse the above ingredients in boiling water and drink as tea.

Effect

Relieves convulsions, induces resuscitation, and calms the mind.

Indications

Palpitations and susceptibility to fright.

Source

Ci Xi Guang Xu Yi Fang Xuan Yi

YUAN ROU ER REN CHA

Main Ingredients

Long Yan Rou (Arillus longan)	12 grams
Chao Suan Zao Ren (parched Semen ziziphi spinosae)	12 grams
Chao Bai Zi Ren (parched *Semen platycladi*)	6 grams

Preparation and Administration

Infuse the above ingredients in boiling water and drink as tea.

Effect

Nourishes the heart to calm the mind.

Indications

Palpitations, insomnia, and amnesia (all due to deficiency of the heart-*qi* and heart-blood).

QING XIN DAI CHA YIN

Main Ingredients

Lian Zi Xin (Plumula nelumbinis)	3 grams
Deng Xin (Medulla junci)	3 grams
Zhu Ye (Herba lophatheri)	3 grams

Chao Suan Zao Ren (Parched
Semen ziziphi spinosae)   9 grams

Preparation and Administration

Infuse the above ingredients in boiling water and drink as tea.

Effect

Removes heart-fire and nourishes the heart to calm the mind.

Indications

Palpitations and insomnia due to *yin* deficiency of the heart
and hypertension.

2.5.5 HERBAL TEA FOR PREVENTING AND TREATING COMMON DISEASES

JU ZHA DAI CHA YIN

Main Ingredients

Ju Hua (Flos chrysanthemi)   12 grams
Sheng Shan Zha (fresh Fructus crataegi)   12 grams

Preparation and Administration

Infuse the above ingredients in boiling water and drink as tea.

Effect

Lowers blood pressure, reduces cholesterol levels, and resists
myocardial ischemia.

Indications

Hypertension, hyperlipernia, and coronary heart disease.

SHOU WU JUE MING CHA

Main Ingredients

He Shou Wu (Radix polygoni multiflori)   12 grams
Jue Ming Zi (Semen cassiae)   12 grams

Preparation and Administration

Infuse the above ingredients in boiling water and drink as tea.

Effect

Reduces cholesterol levels and resists atherosclerosis and
myocardial ischemia.

Indications

Hyperlipernia, atherosclerosis, and coronary heart disease
accompanied by constipation.

FU FANG YU MI XU CHA

Main Ingredients

Yu Mi Xu (Stigma maydis)   30 grams
Che Qian Zi (Semen plantaginis)   15 grams
Ze Xie (Rhizoma alismatis)   12 grams

Preparation and Administration

Infuse the above ingredients in boiling water and drink as tea.

Effect

Induces diuresis and lowers blood pressure, blood sugar
concentration, and cholesterol levels.

Indications
Nephritic edema, ascites due to cirrhosis, and hypertension.

Main Ingredients

Wu Long Cha (tea of Wulong type)	6 grams
Ze Xie (Rhizoma alismatis)	12 grams
Sheng Shan Zha (Fructus crataegi)	12 grams
Yi Yi Ren (Semen coicis)	12 grams
Chen Pi (Pericarpium citri reticulatae)	3 grams

Preparation and Administration
Infuse the above ingredients in boiling water and drink as tea.
Effect
Reduces cholesterol levels, induces diuresis, and aids in
weight reduction.
Indications
Those who suffer from simple obesity or hyperlipernia should
take this tea regularly.

Main Ingredients
Tian Qi (Radix notoginseng)
Shan Cha (Camellia)
Bai Pi Gen (Rhizoma imperatae)
Dosage
Tea in pouches, 4.0–4.8 grams in each.
Administration
Take hot after being steeped in boiling water for a moment.
Use one pouch each time, three times daily, the tea of one
pouch can be infused with boiling water 2–3 times.
Effect
Regulates metabolism, promotes lipodieresis, reduces choles-
terol, and activates blood circulation.
Indications
Simple obesity, cardio-cerebral diseases, and disorders of the
elderly.

Main Ingredients

Luo Bu Ma Ye (Foliurn apocyni veneti)	3 grams
Gou Teng (Ramulus uncariae cum uncis)	15 grams
Dan Pi (Cortex moutan)	6 grams

Preparation and Administration
Infuse the above ingredients in boiling water and drink as tea.
Effect
Lowers blood pressure.

Indications

Hypertension, especially that due to hyperactivity of the liver-*Yang*.

Main Ingredients

Huang Qi (Radix astragali)	15 grams
Yu Mi Xu (Stigma maydis)	30 grams
Shi Wei (Folium pyrrosiae)	21 grams

Preparation and Administration

Infuse the above ingredients in boiling water and drink as tea.

Effect

Invigorates *qi* and promotes diuresis. Patients with proteinuria due to nephritis will have the protein and edema reduced to a certain extent if they take this tea regularly.

Main Ingredients

Xian He Ye (fresh *Folium nelumbinis*)	one piece
Pei Lan (Herba eupatorii)	6 grams
Huo Xiang (Herba agastachis)	6 grams
Ju Hua (Flos chrysanthemi)	6 grams
Jin Yin Hua (Flos lonicerae)	6 grams

Preparation and Administration

Infuse the above ingredients in boiling water and drink as tea.

Effect

Clears away summer-heat and summer-dampness.

Usage

Prevention of heatstroke.

Main Ingredients

Gan Jiang (Rhizoma zingiberis)	6 grams
Liang Jiang (Rhizoma alpiniae officinarum)	3 grams
Chen Pi (Pericarpium citri reticulatae)	3 grams
Wu Zhu Yu (Fructus evodiae)	1.5 grams
Ding Xiang (Flos caryophylli)	1.5 grams

Preparation and Administration

Infuse the above ingredients in boiling water and drink as tea.

Effect

Warms the middle *jiao*, dispels cold, and relieves pain.

Indications

Pain in the stomach and abdomen, hiccups, and vomiting due to stomach-cold.

JIAN WEI CHA

Main Ingredients

Xu Chang Qing (Radix cynanchi paniculati)	9 grams
Mai Dong (Radix ophiopogonis)	9 grams
Sheng Gan Cao (Radix glycyrrhizae)	6 grams
Ju Hong (Exocarpium citri reticulatae)	4.5 grams
Mei Gui Hua (Flos rosae rugosae)	1.5 grams

Preparation and Administration

Infuse the above ingredients in boiling water and drink as tea.

Notes

According to the report written by Gao Shujun and issued in the ninth issue of the *Journal of New Traditional Chinese Medicine*, 1981, this herbal tea was administered to treat superficial and atrophic antral gastritis with the total effective rate reaching 90.98% and the obvious effective rate 44.26%.

QING JIE CHA

Main Ingredients

Jin Yin Hua (Flos lonicerae)	12 grams
Ju Hua (Flos chrysanthemi)	12 grams
Bo He (Herba menthae)	6 grams
Sheng Gan Cao (Radix glycyrrhizae)	6 grams
Huang Lian (Rhizoma coptidis)	3 grams
Zhu Ye (Herba lophatheri)	3 grams

Preparation and Administration

Infuse the above ingredients in boiling water and drink as tea.

Effect

Removes heat and toxic substances.

Indications

Prevention and treatment of furuncles, boils, congestion, and swelling, as well as pain in the eyes due to toxic heat.

2.6 Medicated Gruel for Healthcare

Medicated gruel for healthcare is a thin porridge prepared by cooking selected Chinese drugs together with rice or millet and certain condiments under the guidance of the theories of TCM. It is used to treat diseases. Taking medicated gruel is an important method of protecting health.

The Chinese have long since used medicated gruel prepared by cooking rice or millet and Chinese drugs to treat diseases. The earliest records of which may be traced to the book, *Shi Ji Bian Que Cang Gong Lie Zhuan*, written by Si Ma Qian during the Han dynasty and to 14 kinds of medical books unearthed from the Han Tombs at Mawangdui, Hunan Province. During the Tang and Song dynasties, there was a great development in medicated gruel therapy, which was widely used at that time by physicians and common people to treat and prevent diseases. During the Yuan dynasty, the publications of the book, *Yin Shan Zheng Yao*, written by Hu Sihui and the book, *Shou Qin Yang Lao Xin Shu*, written by Zhou Xuan made contributions to the development of health preservation with medicated gruel. Since the Ming and Qing dynasties, medicated gruel therapy has further developed and has become a systematic therapy for curing diseases, strengthening health, and prolonging life.

Medicated gruel can be used as a means to prevent diseases and as an adjuvant for acute diseases. It may be administered either for recuperation or during illness. Taking it is indeed a good way for middle-aged and elderly people to keep fit. Medicated gruel may be prepared by cooking rice or millet with crude or finely powdered drugs, original juice of drugs, or decoction of drugs.

Different medicated gruels are composed of various ingredients. They invigorate and enrich blood, restore *yang*, and nourish *yin*.

REN SHEN ZHOU

Main Ingredients

Ren Shen (*Radix ginseng* powdered)	3 grams
Bing Tang (crystal sugar)	small amount
Jing Mi (*Semen oryzae sativae*)	100 grams

Preparation
Cook the powder of *Ren Shen* and *Jing Mi* into gruel in a clay pot. When the gruel is almost done, add crystal sugar to it.

Effect
Invigorates primordial *qi*, tonifies the five *zang* organs, and prevents aging.

Indications
All the disorders due to the deficiency of *qi*, blood, and body fluids; deficiency and weakness of the five *zang* organs; emaciation due to long-lasting diseases; poor appetite; chronic diarrhea; palpitations; shortness of breath; insomnia; amnesia; and sexual hypofunction.

Administration
Take on an empty stomach in the morning during autumn or winter.

Caution
This gruel should not be prepared in an iron vessel. In the course of treatment, radish and tea are to be avoided.

Notes
3 grams of *Ren Shen* in the prescription may be substituted by 15 grams of *Dang Shen* (*Radix codonopsis*).

Source
Shi Jian Ben Cao

Main Ingredients

Zhi Huang Qi (Radix astragali praeparata)	30–60 grams
Ren Shen (Radix ginseng)	3–5 grams
Bai Tang (white sugar)	small amount
Jing Mi (Semen oryzae sativae)	100–150 grams

Preparation

Cut *Ren Shen* and *Huang Qi* into thin slices, and steep them in cold water in a clay pot for half an hour. Bring the contents to the boil, and maintain the boil on a lower heat until a concentrated decoction is made. Filter the decoction and cook the drugs in the same way for the second decoction. Mix the two decoctions and divide the mixture into two portions. Place either portion, *Jing Mi*, and an appropriate amount of water into a pot and heat the pot in the morning or evening. At the time when the gruel is nearly ready, add *Bai Tang* to it.

Effect

Invigorates vital *qi*, cures consumptive diseases, strengthens the spleen and stomach, and prevents senility.

Indications

Syndrome due to the deficiency of *qi* and blood, indicated by internal injury due to overstrain, weak physiques in the elderly, spontaneous sweating due to debility, poor appetite, and general edema.

Administration

Take the gruel in the morning or evening for 3–5 days. You should allow 2–3 days between courses.

Caution

In the course of treatment, radish and tea are to be avoided.

Notes

Ren Shen may be ground into fine powder, which is put into the gruel and cooked.

Source

Sheng Ji Zong Lu

Main Ingredients

Da Zao (Fructus jujubae)	10–15 dates
Jing Mi (Semen oryzae sativae)	100 grams

Preparation

Cook the two ingredients into gruel in regular way.

Effect

Invigorates *qi* and blood and strengthens the spleen and stomach.

Indications

Poor appetite due to deficiency of the stomach in the elderly, loose stools due to deficiency of the spleen, *qi* and blood, anemia, chronic hepatitis, malnutrition, and body weakness after illness.

Administration

Take as light refreshments or as a food at breakfast or supper.

Caution

This gruel should not be used by those that are obese, middle-aged, or elderly and that have the syndrome of abundant phlegm-dampness.

Source

Sheng Ji Zong Lu

SHEN LING ZHOU

Main Ingredients

Ren Shen (Radix ginseng)	3–5 grams
Bai Fu Ling (Poria)	15–20 grams
Sheng Jiang (Rhizoma zingiberis recens)	3–5 grams
Jing Mi (Semen oryzae sativae)	100 grams

Preparation

Cut *Ren Shen* and *Sheng Jiang* into slices and pound *Fu Ling* into particles, and decoct the slices and particles in water. Cook the decoction and *Jing Mi* into gruel.

Effect

Restores and invigorates *qi* and nourishes the spleen and stomach.

Indications

Qi deficiency of the spleen and stomach, listlessness, poor appetite, regurgitation, and loose stools.

Administration

This gruel should be eaten warm on an empty stomach in the morning and evening intermittently year round.

Notes

15 grams of *Dang Shen* (*Radix codonopsis*) may be used to substitute for *Ren Shen.*

Source

Sheng Ji Zong Lu

SHAN YAO ZHOU

Main Ingredients

Shan Yao (Rhizoma dioscoreae)	45–60 grams
Jing Mi (Semen oryzae sativae)	100–150 grams

Preparation

Clean *Shan Yao* and cut it into slices. Cook the slices and *Jing Mi* into a gruel.

Effect

Invigorates the spleen and stomach and nourishes the lung and kidneys.

Indications

Hypofunction of the spleen and stomach, chronic diarrhea, cough and asthma due to overstrain, poor appetite, listlessness, diabetes, and chronic nephritis.

Administration

This gruel may be eaten hot in the morning and evening all the year round.

Notes

If *Xian Shan Yao* (fresh *Rhizoma dioscoreae*) is used, its dose should be 100–120 grams

Source

Sa Qian Zhai Jing Yan Fang

BAI BIAN DOU ZHOU

Main Ingredients

Chao Bai Bian Dou (parched *Semen dolichoris album*)	60 grams
Jing Mi (Semen oryzae sativae)	100 grams

Preparation

Cook the two above ingredients into gruel with *Bai Bian Dou* until it is well done.

Effect

Invigorates the spleen and stomach, clears away summer-heat, and arrests diarrhea.

Indications

Deficiency of the spleen and stomach, poor appetite, vomiting, chronic diarrhea, dysentery due to summer-dampness, restlessness and thirst in summer.

Administration

Take at breakfast and supper in summer and autumn.

Notes

If *Xian Bai Bian Dou* (fresh *Semen dolichoris album*) is used, its dose should be 120 grams

Source

Yan Nian Mi Zhi

HUANG QI ZHOU

Main Ingredients

Sheng Huang Qi (Radix astragali)	30–60 grams
Jing Mi (Semen Oryzae sativae)	100 grams
Chen Pi (Pericarpium citri reticulatae powdered)	1 gram
Hong Tang (brown sugar)	small amount

Preparation

Decoct *Huang Qi* in water and concentrate it. Cook the concentration together with *Jing Mi* and *Hong Tang*. When the gruel is almost done, add the powder of *Chen Pi* to it.

Effect

Invigorates primordial *qi*, strengthens the spleen and stomach, and induces diuresis to alleviate edema.

Indications

Disorders due to the deficiency of *qi* and blood, chronic

diarrhea, spontaneous sweating due to weak physique, senile edema, chronic hepatitis, chronic nephritis, and ulcers.

Administration

Take hot at breakfast and supper.

Caution

This gruel is not for patients with the syndrome of *yin* deficiency.

Source

Leng Lu Yi Hua

LUO HUA SHENG ZHOU

Main Ingredients

Luo Hua Sheng (Semen arachidis hypogaeae with the red coat)	45 grams
Jing Mi (Semen oryzae sativae)	100 grams
Bing Tang (crystal sugar)	proper amount
Huai Shan Yao (Rhizoma dioscoreae)	30 grams

Preparation

Wash *Hua Sheng* and break it up. Cut *Shan Yao* into slices. Cook the broken *Hua Sheng Jing Mi* and the sliced *Shan Yao* together. Before the gruel is cooked, add *Bing Tang* to it.

Effect

Strengthens the spleen to induce appetite and promote digestion, moistens the lungs, arrests coughs, and nourishes the blood to activate lactation.

Indications

Unproductive cough due to dryness of the lungs, regurgitation due to deficiency of the spleen, anemia, and postpartum hypolactation.

Administration

This gruel may be eaten over a long period of time.

Caution

15 grams of *Bai He* may be used instead of *Shan Yao*. In the process of cooking, the red skin of peanuts should be retained. Over-intake of this gruel is contraindicated in patients suffering from diarrhea.

Source

Zhou Pu

ZHU YU ER BAO ZHOU

Main Ingredients

Shan Yao (Rhizoma dioscoreae)	60 grams
Sheng Yi Yi Ren (Semen coicis)	60 grams
Shi Bing (dried persimmon)	30 grams

Preparation

Cook *Yi Yi Ren* until it is well done. Pound *Shan Yao* and cut *Shi Bing* into small pieces. Cook them together with *Yi Yi Ren* until they are well done.

Effect

Invigorates the lungs, strengthens the spleen, and nourishes the stomach.

Indications

Disorders due to *qi* deficiency of the spleen and lungs, such as internal heat due to deficiency of *yin*, dry cough, loose stool, and poor appetite.

Administration

This gruel is mainly used for those recuperating from chronic diseases. It is to be taken twice daily. One course of treatment is 5–7 days.

Notes

In this gruel, *Shan Yao* is used as a substitute for *Jing Mi* (Semen Oryzae sativae).

Source

Yi Xue Zhong Zhong Can Xi Lu

NUO MI E JIAO ZHOU

Main Ingredients

E Jiao (Colla corii asini)	30 grams
Nuo Mi (Semen oryzae glutinosae)	100 grams
Hong Tang (brown sugar)	small amount

Preparation

Cook *Nuo Mi*. Before it is done, add *E Jiao* that has been pounded into small pieces. Continue cooking, and keep stirring the contents for 2–3 minutes. Then add the brown sugar, thus obtaining the gruel.

Effect

Nourishes *yin,* supplements blood, enriches blood, prevents miscarriages, and replenishes the lungs.

Indications

Deficiency of blood, cough due to consumptive diseases, long-lasting cough with hemoptysis, hematochezia and hypomenorrhea due to deficiency of blood, metrostaxis, threatened abortion, and vaginal bleeding during pregnancy.

Administration

This gruel can be eaten intermittently. One course of treatment is three days.

Caution

Consumption of this gruel by those with the syndrome of deficiency of the spleen and stomach is not advisable.

Source

Shi Yi Xin Jian

Main Ingredients

Long Yan Rou (Arillus longan)	15 grams
Hong Zao (Fructus jujubae)	3–5 grams
Jing Mi (Semen oryzae sativae)	100 grams
Bai Tang (white sugar)	small amount

Preparation

Combine and cook the above ingredients into gruel. Sugar may be added to taste.

Effect

Tonifies the heart, relieves mental strain, benefits the spleen, and nourishes the blood.

Indications

Disorders due to deficiency of the heart-blood, such as palpitation, insomnia, poor memory, anemia, and diarrhea due to deficiency of the spleen, edema, and weak physique.

Administration

Take hot and in a limited amount each time.

Caution

This gruel is not advisable for those that are ill with common cold of wind-cold type marked by aversion to cold, fever, and a thick, greasy tongue coating .

Source

Lao Lao Heng Yan

Main Ingredients

He Shou Wu (Radix polygoni multiflori)	30–60 grams
Jing Mi (Semen oryzae sativae)	100 grams
Hong Zao (Fructus jujubae)	3–5 dates
Hong Tang (brown sugar)	small amount

Preparation

Decoct He Shou Wu in water and concentrate the decoction. Place the decoction in a clay pot and cook together with Jing Mi and Hong Zao. Add Hong Tang when the gruel is nearly done, and continue the cooking for 1–2 minutes.

Effect

Invigorates qi and blood and replenishes the liver and kidneys.

Indications

Deficiency of the liver and kidneys, early graying of hair, dizziness and tinnitus due to deficiency of blood, soreness and weakness of the loins and knees, constipation, hypertension, coronary heart disease, and hyperlipemia.

Administration

One course of treatment is 7–10 days in length, twice daily. Allow a five day interval between every two courses.

Source

Zun Sheng Ba Jian

Caution

This gruel should not be prepared in an iron pot. During the course of treatment, scallions and garlic should be avoided. Additionally, this gruel should not be taken by those suffering from diarrhea.

Main Ingredients

Niu Ru (cow's milk)	an appropriate amount
Da Mi (rice)	100 grams
Bai Tang (white sugar)	small amount

Preparation

Cook the rice until it is nearly cooked. Add the milk and sugar, and finish cooking.

Effect

Restores *qi* and strengthens the spleen and stomach.

Indications

All the consumptive diseases, deficiency of *qi* and blood, emaciation after an illness or childbirth, senile weakness, and malnourished infants.

Administration

Eat hot on an empty stomach in the morning and evening

Caution

Yang Ru (milk from ewe) may be used instead of *Niu Ru*. If this gruel is prepared for infants, *Ren Ru* (human milk) should be used. In summer, the milk must be kept fresh.

Source

Qu Xian Shen Yin

Main Ingredients

Hai Shen (sea cucumber)	an appropriate amount
Jing Mi (Semen oryzae sativae)	100 grams

Preparation

Soak *Hai Shen* with water to soften and clean it, cut it into pieces, and boil it thoroughly. Cook it together with *Jing Mi* into gruel.

Effect

Tonifies the kidneys, replenishes vital essence, and nourishes blood.

Indications

Deficiency of vital essence and blood, weak constitution, sexual hypofunction, seminal emission, and frequent urination.

Administration

This gruel may be regularly taken on an empty stomach in the morning. The course of treatment is determined according to need.

Caution

Nuo Mi (*Semen oryzae glutinosae*) may be used instead of *Jing Mi*.

Source
Lao Lao Heng Yan

Main Ingredients

Sang Shen (Fructus mori)	20–30 grams
Nuo Mi (Semen oryzae glutinosae)	100 grams
Bing Tang (crystal sugar)	small amount

Preparation

Steep *Sang Shen* in water for a few minutes and then clean it. Cook it together with *Nuo Mi* into gruel in a clay pot. Before the gruel is completely cooked, add *Bing Tang.*

Effect

Tonifies the liver and kidneys, nourishes blood, and improves eyesight.

Indications

Yin deficiency of the liver and kidneys, dizziness, blurred vision, soreness and weakness of the loins and knees, early graying of hair, and constipation due to dryness in the intestines.

Administration

Eat regularly on an empty stomach.

Caution

This gruel should not be taken by those suffering from diarrhea and should not be prepared in an iron pot. If *Xian Sang Shen* (fresh *Fructus mori*) is used instead of the dried, the dosage should be 30–60 grams.

Source
Zhou Pu

Main Ingredients

Mu Ji (a hen)	weighing 1500–2000 grams
Jing Mi (Semen oryzae sativae)	100 grams

Preparation

Clean the hen, and boil it in water to get concentrated soup. Divide the soup into several portions. Use each portion to cook with *Jing Mi* into gruel.

Effect

Nourishes the five *zang* organs and invigorates *qi* and the blood.

Administration

Should be taken hot.

Caution

This gruel should be not be taken by patients with fever.

Source
Zhong Guo Peng Ren

Main Ingredients

Tu Si Zi (Semen cuscutae)	30–60 grams
Jing Mi (Semen oryzae sativae)	100 grams
Bai Tang (white sugar)	an appropriate amount

Preparation

Clean *Tu Si Zi* and pound it into small pieces. Decoct it in water. Cook the decoction and *Jing Mi* into gruel. When the gruel is almost cooked, add sugar to taste.

Effect

Tonifies the kidneys to replenish vital essence and nourishes the liver to improve eyesight.

Indications

Deficiency of the liver and kidneys, soreness and weakness of the loins and knees, impotence, seminal emission, premature ejaculation, dizziness, tinnitus, and frequent urination.

Administration

Take in the morning and evening and for a long time.

Caution

If *Xian Tu Si Zi* (fresh *Semen cuscutae*) is used instead of the dried, the dosage should be 69–100 grams.

Source

Zhou Pu

Main Ingredients

Rou Cong Rong (Herba Cistanchis)	10–15 grams
Jing Yang Rou (fine mutton)	100 grams
Jing Mi (Semen oryzae sativae)	100 grams
Xi Yan (refined salt)	small amount
Cong Bai (Bulbus allii fistulosi)	2 pieces
Sheng Jiang (Rhizoma zingiberis recens)	3 slices

Preparation

Wash *Rou Cong Rong* and *Jing Yang Rou*. Clean and cut them into small pieces separately. Decoct *Rou Cong Rong* in a clay pot. Cook the decoction together with *Jing Yang Rou* and *Jing Mi*. After the contents boil, *Xi Yan*, *Cong Bai* and *Sheng Jiang* are added. Continue to cook until the gruel is done.

Effect

Invigorates the kidney-*yang*, strengthens the spleen and stomach, and loosens the bowels to relieve constipation.

Indications

Deficiency of the kidney-*yang*, impotence, seminal emission, premature ejaculation, cold-pain in the loins and knees, infertility due to coldness of the womb, emaciation and weakness of the body, internal injury due to overstrain, insufficiency of the spleen-*yang*, and constipation in the elderly.

Administration

One course of treatment is 5–7 days. This gruel should be taken in winter.

Caution

This gruel is avoided during the summer and by those suffering from diarrhea or sexual hyperfunction. It must not be prepared in an iron pot.

Source

Ben Cao Gang Mu

HU TAO ZHOU

Main Ingredients

Hu Tao Ren (Semen juglandis)	10–15 grams
Jing Mi (Semen oryzae sativae)	100 grams

Preparation

Pound *Hu Tao Ren* and cook it together with *Jing Mi* into gruel.

Effect

Tonifies the kidneys, reinforces the lungs, and moistens the intestines.

Indications

Pain in the waist and weakness of the legs due to deficiency of the kidney, unrelieved cough and shortness of breath due to deficiency of the lung, chronic constipation, debility after recovering from a disease, and urinary tract infection.

Administration

Take as prescribed.

Caution

This gruel should not be used by those who discharge thin stools.

Source

Hai Shang Ji Yan Fang (Hai Shang Ji's Empirical Recipes)

LI ZHI ZHOU

Main Ingredients

Gan Li Zhi (dried *Fructus litchi*)	5–7 fruits
Jing Mi (Semen oryzae sativae)	100 grams

Preparation

Remove the shells of *Gan Li Zhi* to get the pulp; cook in water together with *Jing Mi* into gruel.

Effect

Warms *yang* and invigorates *qi*, promotes the production of body fluids, and nourishes the blood.

Indications

Diarrhea due to deficiency of *yang*, diarrhea before dawn, and halitosis.

Administration

This gruel is to be eaten at supper. One course of treatment is 3–5 days in length.

Caution

Those who have hyperactivity of fire due to deficiency of *yin* should avoid this gruel. *Nuo Mi* (*Semen oryzae glutinosae*) can be used to substitute for *Jing Mi*.

Source

Quan Zhou Ben Cao

LI ZI ZHOU

Main Ingredients

Li Zi (chestnuts)	10–15 nuts
Jing Mi (*Semen oryzae sativae*)	100 grams

Preparation

Remove the shells of *Li Zi* and cook it with *Jing Mi* into gruel.

Effect

Tonifies the kidneys, strengthens muscles and tendons, and invigorates the spleen and stomach.

Indications

Infirmity with age, pain of the loins due to deficiency of the kidney, weakness of the legs, and diarrhea due to deficiency of the spleen.

Administration

Take at breakfast and supper all year round.

Caution

30 grams of *Li Fen* (powder of chestnut) may be used to substitute for 10–15 chestnuts and *Nuo Mi* (*Semen oryzae glutirosae*) may be used to replace *Jing Mi*.

Source

Ben Cao Gang Mu

Que Er Yao Zhou

Main Ingredients

Ma Que (sparrow)	5 sparrows
Tu Si Zi (*Semen cuscutae*)	30–45 grams
Fu Pen Zi (*Fructus rubi*)	10–15 grams
Gou Qi Zi (*Fructus lycii*)	20–30 grams
Jing Mi (*Semen oryzae sativae*)	100 grams
Xi Yan (fine salt)	small amount
Cong Bai (*Bulbus allii Fistulosi*)	2 pieces
Sheng Jiang (*Rhizoma Zingiberis Recens*)	3 slices

Preparation

Decoct *Tu Si Zi*, *Fu Pen Zi*, and *Gou Qi Zi* in a clay pot. Bake in wine the plucked and cleaned *Ma Que*. Finally, cook the prepared *Ma Que* and *Jing Mi* together in water into a gruel. When the gruel is almost cooked add *Xi Yan*, *Cong Bai*, and *Sheng Jiang* and finish cooking.

Effect

Strengthens *yang*, replenishes vital essence and the blood, tonifies the liver and kidneys, and warms the loins and knees.

Indications

Deficiency of the kidney-*qi*, cold-soreness of the loins and knees, impotence, premature ejaculation, seminal emission, dizziness, tinnitus, profuse and clear urine, and irregular leukorrhea.

Administration

This gruel is to be taken in winter. One course of treatment is 3–5 days in length.

Caution

This gruel should be avoided by those that have fever or sexual hyperfunction.

Source

Tai Ping Sheng Hui Fang

LU JIAO JIAO ZHOU

Main Ingredients

Lu Jiao Jiao (Colla cornus cervi)	15–20 grams
Jing Mi (Semen oryzae sativae)	100 grams
Sheng Jiang (Rhizoma zingiberis recens)	3 slices

Preparation

Cook *Jing Mi* alone in water. When the content boils, add *Lu Jiao Jiao* and *Sheng Jiang,* and finish cooking the gruel.

Effect

Tonifies the kidney-*yang*, and replenishes vital essence and the blood.

Indications

Deficiency of the kidney-*qi*, emaciation due to consumptive diseases, impotence, seminal emission, premature ejaculation, infertility due to cold womb, metrorrhagia, metrostaxis, and irregular leukorrhea.

Administration

This gruel is to be taken during the winter. One course of treatment is 3–5 days in length.

Caution

This gruel should not be prescribed in summer and should not be used by those that have hyperactivity of fire due to deficiency of *yin* or fever.

Source

Ben Cao Gang Mu

Gou Qi Yang Shen Zhou

Main Ingredients

Gou Qi Ye (Folium lycii)	250 grams
Xian Yang Shen (fresh sheep kidney)	a whole one
Yang Rou (mutton)	100 grams
Jing Mi (Semen oryzae sativae)	100–150 grams
Cong Bai (Bulbus allii fistulosi)	2 pieces
Xi Yan (fine salt)	small amount

Preparation

Wash *Xian Yang Shen*. Remove the membrane and cut the *Xian Yan Shen* into small pieces. Wash *Yang Rou* and clean and cut it into small pieces as well. Decoct *Gou Qi Ye* in water. Cook the decoction with the small pieces of *Yang Shen* and Yang *Rou*, the *Jing Mi* and the *Cong Bai* together into gruel. Before the gruel is fully cooked, add *Xi Yan*.

Effect

Replenishes the kidney-*yin*, tonifies the kidney-*qi*, and reinforces the kidney-*yang*.

Indications

Internal injury due to kidney deficiency, soreness and weakness of the loins and knees, dizziness, tinnitus, sexual hypofunction, and deficiency of *yang*.

Administration

Take in winter.

Caution

This gruel should not be used by those who are of *yang*-excess type. *Gou Qi Zi* (*Semen lycii*) may be used to replace *Gou Qi Ye*.

Source

Yin Shan Zheng Yao

SHAN YU ROU ZHOU

Main Ingredients

Shan Yu Rou (Fructus corni)	15–20 grams
Jing Mi (Semen oryzae sativae)	100 grams
Bai Tang (white sugar)	an appropriate amount

Preparation

Wash *Shan Yu Rou*. Clean and remove its pits, and cook it together with *Jing Mi* in a clay pot. When the gruel is almost prepared, add *Bai Tang*.

Effect

Tonifies the liver and kidneys, controls nocturnal emissions, and sweating.

Indications

Deficiency of the liver and kidney, dizziness, blurred vision, tinnitus, soreness of the loins, incessant sweating due to debility, seminal emission, and enuresis.

Administration

One course of treatment is 3–5 days in length.

Caution

This gruel should not be taken again once the disease is cured. It should not be taken by those suffering from a fever.

Source

Zhou Pu

YU ZHU ZHOU

Main Ingredients

Yu Zhu (Rhizoma polygonati odorati)	15–20 grams
Jing Mi (Semen oryzae sativae)	100 grams
Bing Tang (crystal sugar)	small amount

Preparation

Decoct *Yu Zhu* in water and concentrate the decoction. Mix the concentrated decoction with *Jing Mi* and cook them in an appropriate amount of water into thin gruel. Before the gruel is finished cooking, add *Bing Tang*, and continue cooking for another 1–2 minutes.

Effect

Nourishes *yin*, moistens the lungs, and promotes the production of body fluids to relieve coughs.

Indications

Deficiency of the lung-*yin*, dry cough with less or no sputum due to dryness of the lungs, and fever due to deficiency of *yin*. Taking this gruel may be treated as an accessory therapy for various heart diseases and cardiac functional insufficiencies.

Administration

Take in the morning and evening. One course of treatment is 5–7 days in length.

Caution

This gruel should not be taken by those suffering from syndrome of phlegm retained, of *qi* stagnated in the stomach, or of indigestion. If *Xian Yu Zhu* (fresh *Rhizoma polygonati odorati*) is used instead of the dried, the dosage should be 30–60 grams.

Source

Zhou Pu

TIAN MEN DONG ZHOU

Main Ingredients

Tian Dong (Radix asparagi)	15–20 grams
Jing Mi (Semen oryzae sativae)	90–100 grams
Bing Tang (crystal sugar)	small amount

Preparation

Decoct *Tian Men Dong* in water and concentrate the decoction. Cook the decoction with *Jing Hi* into a gruel. When the gruel is almost done, add *Bing Tang*.

Effect

Nourishes *yin*, moistens the lungs, and promotes the production of body fluids to relieve cough.

Indications

Deficiency of the kidney-*yin*, excess heat in the interior due to deficiency of *yin*, dry mouth due to absence of body fluids or the deficiency of the lung-*yin*, and night sweating.

Administration

One course of treatment is 3–5 days in length. There should be a 3-day interval between every two courses.

Caution

This gruel is contraindicated for those who are suffering from diarrhea and cold due to being attacked by exogenous wind-cold.

Source

Yin Shi Bian Lu

SHA SHEN ZHOU

Main Ingredients

Sha Shen (Radix adenophorae)	15–30 grams
Jing Mi (Semen oryzae sativae)	100 grams
Bing Tang (crystal sugar)	an appropriate amount

Preparation

Decoct *Sha Shen* in water. Cook the decoction with *Jing Mi* into gruel. When the gruel is almost cooked, add *Bing Tang.*

Effect

Moistens the lungs, nourishes the stomach, and removes phlegm to arrest coughs.

Indications

Dry cough with little sputum due to dryness of the lungs or long-standing unproductive cough due to deficiency of lung-*qi.* Also *yin* deficiency of the lungs and stomach, dry throat, or thirst due to the exhaustion of body fluid by febrile diseases.

Administration

Take as prescribed.

Caution

This gruel should be cooked thin. It should not be taken by those who suffer the symptom of cough due to wind-cold.

Source

Zhou Pu

BAI HE FEN ZHOU

Main Ingredients

Bai He Fen (*Bulbus lihi* in the form of powder)	30 grams
Jing Mi (Semen Oryzae Sativae)	100 grams
Bing Tang (crystal sugar)	an appropriate amount

Preparation

Cook *Bai He Fen* and *Jing Mi* together into gruel. When the gruel is almost cooked, add *Bing Tang.*

Effect

Moistens the lungs to relieve cough, and nourishes the heart to calm the mind.

Indications

Senility, chronic bronchitis, cough due to heat or dryness in the lung, residual fever in the late stage of febrile diseases, and menopausal syndrome.

Administration

Take as prescribed.

Caution

This gruel should not be taken by those who suffer with the symptom of cough due to wind-cold or the syndrome of cold of the deficiency type in the spleen and stomach. If *Xian Bai He* (fresh *Bulbus lilii*) is used, the dosage should be 60 grams.

Source

Ben Cao Gang Mu

LIAN ZI FEN ZHOU

Main Ingredients

Lian Zi Fen (*Semen nelumbinis* in the form of powder)	15–20 grams
Jing Mi (Semen oryzae savitae)	100 grams

Preparation

Cook *Lian Zi* until it is done. Peel it, dry it, and grind it into powder, and cook it together with *Jing Mi* into gruel.

Effect

Nourishes the heart to calm the mind, replenishes the kidneys, tonifies the spleen, and prevents aging.

Indications

Infirmity with age, insomnia or dream-disturbed sleep, chronic diarrhea, and frequent urination at night.

Caution

This gruel should not be taken by those suffering from the symptom of fever due to cold or the symptom of constipation.

Source

Tai Ping Sheng Hui Fang

SUAN ZAO REN ZHOU

Main Ingredients

Suan Zao Ren (Semen ziziphi spinosae)	30–40 grams
Jing Mi (Semen oryzae sativae)	100 grams

Preparation

Crush *Suan Zao Ren* and decoct it in water. Cook *Jing Mi* in an appropriate amount of water. When *Jing Mi* is half done, add the decoction to it, and continue the cooking until the gruel is cooked.

Effect

Nourishes the liver, relieves mental stress, calms the mind, and arrests sweating.

Indications

Neurosism, insomnia, severe palpitations spontaneous sweating, and night sweating.

Administration
Take hot at supper.
Notes
Either prepared or unprepared *Suan Zao Ren* may be used.
Source
Tai Ping Sheng Hui Fang

SHAN ZHA ZHOU

Main Ingredients

Shan Zha (Fructus crataegi)	30–40 g
Jing Mi (Semen oryzae sativae)	100 g
Sha Tang (granulated sugar)	10 g

Preparation
Decoct *Shan Zha* in a clay pot. Then cook together with *Jing Mi* and *Sha Tang* into gruel.
Effect
Strengthens the spleen and stomach, promotes digestion, and disperses blood stasis.
Regular intake of this gruel by the elderly can prevent diseases and strengthen the body.
Indications
Retention of food, abdominal pain, diarrhea, postpartum pain caused by stasis of blood, lochiorrhea, dysmenorrhea, hypertension, coronary heart disease, and hyperlipemia.
Administration
This gruel is to be eaten as light refreshments at breakfast, lunch, and supper. One course of treatment is 7–10 days in length.
Caution
This gruel should not be used by those who suffer from the syndrome of deficiency of the spleen and stomach. If *Xian Shan Zha* (fresh *Fructus crataegi*) is used the dosage should be 60 grams.
Source
Zhou Pu

YI YI REN ZHOU

Main Ingredients

Yi Yi Ren Fen (Semen coicis) in the form of powder	30–60 grams
Jing Mi (Semen orvzae sativae)	100 grams

Preparation
Wash *Yi Yi Ren* and dry it in the sun. Grind it into fine powder, and cook it with *Jing Mi* into gruel.
Effect
Strengthens the spleen and stomach, induces diuresis, and resists tumors.

Indications
Senility edema, spasm of the muscles and tendons, and numbness and pain due to wind-dampness.
Administration
Eat hot at breakfast and supper.
Source
Guang Ji Fang

2.7 Medicated Cake for Healthcare

Cake is a kind of common food that is made by steaming or baking the paste of powdered rice, wheat, or beans. It is soft, easy to digest, and popular among the Chinese people.

Medicated cake is a delicious food and it serves as a product for healthcare in dietotherapy because it contains herbal medicines.

Medicated cakes are usually used to help treat senile and infantile patients with chronic disorders of the spleen and stomach, to help recuperating patients, and to assist those who want to treat and prevent disease.

Taking medicated cakes is a convenient, practical, and self-health-preserving method. This is because most medicines contained in the cakes are mild in nature and because the cakes can be easily made at home. The medicated cakes introduced below are for the most part selected from relevant literature. The introductions and analyses have been enriched with the author's modern knowledge and experience. The prescriptions without the indicated sources are those created by the author.

YANG CHUN BAI XUE GAO

Main Ingredients

Bai Fu Ling (Poria)	150 grams
Huai Shan Yao (Rhizoma dioscoreae)	150 grams
Qian Shi Ren (Semen euryales)	150 grams
Lian Zi Rou (Semen nelumbinis)	150 grams
Chen Cang Mi (long-stored rice)	300 grams
Nuo Mi (Semen Oryzae glutinosae)	300 grams
Bai Sha Tang (white granulated sugar)	900 grams

Preparation
Grind *Bai Fu Ling* with its skin removed with *Huai Shan Yao*, *Qian Shi Ren*, and *Lian Zi Rou* (with the plumule and skin removed) into fine powder. Steam the powder, *Chen Cang Mi*, and *Nuo Mi* together until they are well done. Thoroughly, mix the well-done ingredients with *Bai Sha Tang*, and knead the mixture with water into a paste. Make the paste into cakes. Dry the cakes in the sun, and then store them for use.

Administration
These cakes can be eaten freely by men, women, and children.
Effect
Strengthens the spleen, nourishes the stomach, replenishes
the kidney, and tonifies the heart.
Indications
General debility, dysfunction of the spleen and stomach,
listlessness, and poor appetite.
Notes
This cake is most suitable for the elderly.
Source
Shou Shi Bao Yuan written by Gong Tingxian, a medical official
of the Institute of Imperial Physicians in the Ming dynasty

MI CHUAN ER XIAN GAO

Main Ingredients

Ren Shen (Radix ginseng)	250 grams
Shan Yao (Rhizoma dioscoreae)	250 grams
Bai Fu Ling (Poria)	250 grams
Qian Shi Ren (Semen euryales)	250 grams
Lian Zi Rou (Semen nelumbinis with the plumule and skin removed)	250 grams
Nuo Mi (Semen oryzae glutinosae)	750 grams
Jing Mi (Semen oryzae sativae)	1750 grams
Feng Mi (Mel)	250 grams
Bai Tang (white sugar)	250 grams

Preparation
Grind *Ren Shen, Shan Yao, Bai Fu Ling, Qian Shi Ren, Lian Zi
Rou, Nuo Mi*, and *Jing Mi* into a fine powder and stir the
powder evenly. Dissolve *Feng Mi* and *Bai Tang* in water, and
mix them with the powder thoroughly. Steam the mixture into
cakes, and bake the cakes in a moderate oven.
Administration
Mi Chuan Er Xian Gao may be eaten as a light refreshment. It
may also be made into powder, which is stored in a porcelain
pot. Every morning, a large spoonful of the powder can be
infused with boiled water and eaten.
Effect
Strengthens the teeth, darkens the hair, invigorates both *yin*
and *yang*, replenishes the kidney-*yin*, and nourishes the spleen
and stomach.
Indications
Same as those of *Yang Chun Bai Xue Gao*.
Notes
Compared with *Yang Chun Bai Xue Gao*, this cake contains one
more ingredient, *Ren Shen*, which enhances the cake's ability
to invigorate primordial *qi* and strengthen its tonifying action.

Source
Fu Shou Jing Gang and the book *Ji Yang Gang Mu* both of which are classics of the Ming dynasty.

JIU XIAN WANG DAO GAO

Main Ingredients

Lian Zi Rou (Semen nelumbinis with the plumule and skin removed)	120 grams
Chao Shan Yao (parched *Rhizoma dioscoreae*)	120 grams
Bai Fu Ling (Poria)	120 grams
Yi Ren (Semen coicis)	120 grams
Chao Mai Ya (parched *Fructus hordei germinatus*)	60 grams
Chao Bai Bian Dou (parched *Semen dolichoris album*)	60 grams
Qian Shi (Semen euryales)	60 grams
Shi Shuang (Pruina kaki)	30 grams
Bai Tang (White sugar)	600 grams
Nuo Mi (Semen oryzae glatinosae)	2500 grams

Preparation
Grind all the ingredients into powder except *Nuo Mi*, which is ground separately. Mix the two kinds of powder with an appropriate amount of water into a paste. Steam the paste until it is done. Cut the steamed paste into pieces, and dry the pieces in the sun.

Administration
Eat with rice soup at will.

Effect
Tranquilizes the mind, strengthens primordial *qi*, invigorates the spleen and stomach, activates the appetite, restores *qi*, promotes the regeneration of tissues, and removes dampness and heat.

Indications
These cakes are advisable for those who are old or have weak constitutions.

Source
Wan Bing Hui Chun written by Gong Tingxian in the Ming dynasty and *Chuan Ya Nei Wai Pian* written by Zhao Xuemin in the Qing dynasty

BA XIAN BAI YUN GAO

Main Ingredients

Gan Shan Yao (dried *Rhizoma diosocreat*)	120 grams
Lian Zi Rou (Semen nelumbinis with the plumule and skin removed)	120 grams
Bai Fu Ling (Poria)	120 grams
Qian Shi Rou (Semen euryales with the plumule and skin removed)	120 grams

Yi Yi Ren (Semen coicis)	120 grams
Bai Shao Yao (Radix paeoniae alba)	60 grams
Bai Zhu (Rhizoma atractylodis macrocephalae)	60 grams
Sha Ren (Fructus amomi)	30 grams
Shang Bai Mi Fan (cooked fine rice)	1000 grams
Nuo Mi (Semen oryzae glutinosae)	750 grams
Bai Sha Tang Shuang (frost of white granulated sugar)	1250 grams

Preparation

Grind the first eight ingredients into a fine powder, and mix the powder with *Shang Bai Mi Fan* and *Nuo Mi* into a well-stirred mixture. Once they are mixed, then add *Bai Sha Tang Shuang*. Steam the mixture into cakes.

Administration

Eat at will.

Effect

Invigorates primordial *qi* and regulates physiological functions.

Source

Ming Yi Xuan Yao Ji Shi Qi Fang

BA XIAN ZAO CHAO GAO

Main Ingredients

Chao Bai Zhu (parched *Rhizoma atractylodis macrocephalae*)	120 grams
Shan Yao (Rhizoma dioscoreae)	120 grams
Zhi Shi (Fructus aurantii immaturus)	60 grams
Bai Fu Ling (Poria)	60 grams
Chao Chen Pi (parched *Pericarpiumcitri reticulatae*)	60 grams
Lian Zi Rou (Semen nelumbinis with the plumule and skin removed)	60 grams
Shan Zha (Fructus crataegi with the core removed)	60 grams
Ren Shen (Radix ginseng)	30 grams
Bai Mi (fine rice)	2750 grams
Nuo Mi (Senien oryzae glutinosae)	750 grams
Feng Mi (honey)	1500 grams

Preparation

Grind the first eight ingredients into fine powder, and then grind *Bai Mi* and *Nuo Mi*. Mix the two powders and *Feng Mi* thoroughly and make the mixture into a paste. Cut the paste into small pieces, and steam the pieces until they are done. Bake the steamed pieces, and store them in a clay pot.

Administration

Eat 3–5 pieces at a time.

Effect

Regulates the function of the spleen and stomach, and treats incessant diarrhea.

Indications

Cakes of this kind may be eaten regularly by middle-aged and old people that suffer from with the symptom of *qi* deficiency of the spleen.

Source

Ji Yang Gang Mu

BA ZHEN GAO

Main Ingredients

Yi Mi (Semen coicis)	90 grams
Qian Shi (Semen euryales)	90 grams
Bian Dou (Semen dolichoris album)	90 grams
Jian Lian (Semen nelumbinis with the plumule and skin removed)	90 grams
Shan Yao (Rhizoma dioscoreae)	90 grams
Dang Shen (Radix codonopsis)	60 grams
Fu Ling (Poria)	60 grams
Bai Zhu (Rhizoma atractylodis macrocephalae)	30 grams
Bai Tang (white sugar)	240 grams
Bai Mi Fen (Powder of white rice)	an appropriate amount

Preparation

Grind the above ingredients except the *Bai Mi Fen* into fine powder. Mix the powder with *Bai Mi Fen* into a mixture and make the mixture into cakes.

Administration

Eat at will, 2–3 times each day.

Effect

Strengthens and nourishes the spleen and stomach.

Indications

Ba Zhen Gao is indicated for those who have a weak constitution and spleen-*qi*.

Caution

Regular intake of *Ba Zhen Gao* tends to result in stagnation of stomach-*qi*.

Source

Qing Tai Yi Tuan Pei Fang

JIAN PI YANG XIN GAO

Main Ingredients

Fu Shen (Poria cum ligno hospite)	60 grams
Lian Zi Rou (Semen nelumbinis with the plumule and skin removed)	60 grams
Shan Yao (Rhizoma dioscoreae)	60 grams
Bai He (Bulbus lihi)	60 grams
Long Yan Rou (Arillus longan)	60 grams
Bai Tang (white sugar)	150 grams
Nuo Mi Fen (powdered *Semen oryzae glutinosae*)	1000 grams

Preparation

Grind the first five ingredients into fine powder. Mix the powder with *Bai Tang* and *Nuo Mi Fen* thoroughly. Steam the mixture into cakes, which may be baked dry for storage.

Administration

Eat at will and regularly.

Effect

Strengthens the spleen, replenishes *qi*, nourishes the heart, calms the mind, tonifies the kidneys, enriches blood, and is good for strengthening both the heart and spleen.

Indications

Deficiency of *qi* and blood in the heart and spleen, listlessness, poor appetite, bad memory, insomnia, palpitations, shortness of breath, and sallow complexion.

Notes

Compared with the above-mentioned medicated cakes, cakes of this kind have the stronger action of nourishing the heart to calm the mind.

HE ZHONG XIAO SHI GAO

Main Ingredients

Fu Ling (Poria)	45 grams
Bai Bian Dou (Semen dolichoris album)	45 grams
Lian Zi Rou (Semen nelumbinis with the plumule and skin removed)	45 grams
Shan Yao (Rhizoma dioscoreae)	45 grams
Chao Shan Zha (parched *Fructus crataegi*)	45 grams
Chao Mai Ya (parched *Fructus hordei germinatus*)	45 grams
Chao Gu Ya (parched *Fructus oryzae germinatus*)	45 grams
Sha Ren (Fructus amomi)	9 grams
Bai Tang (white sugar)	150 grams
Mi Fen (powder of rice)	1000 grams

Preparation

Grind the first eight ingredients into fine powder. Mix the powder with *Bai Tang* and *Mi Fen* thoroughly, and steam the mixture into cakes. The cakes may be cut into pieces, which are then baked dry.

Administration

Eat at will and regularly.

Effect

Invigorates the spleen and stomach, replenishes *qi*, regulates the stomach to promote digestion, and activates the flow of *qi*.

Indications

Deficiency of the spleen and stomach, poor appetite, abdominal distention, stuffiness and fullness in the epigastrium and abdomen, and food retention.

Notes

Cakes of this kind have both tonifying and resolving effects.

2.8 Medicated Pancakes for Healthcare

Medicated pancakes are also a kind of conventional drug that is used in TCM. Medicated pancakes are made from traditional Chinese drugs in the form of a fine powder, wheat flour, bean flour, or rice flour, sometimes with dates or sugar and oil. They are made by steaming, baking, or frying. Such pancakes are easy to make, convenient to take, delicious, and effective. Medicated pancakes are mild in nature and slow in drug action. This means that only constant administration of them will obtain the prescribed results.

The following are some medicated pancake recipes that are used to prevent diseases, build up health, and prolong life. The prescriptions with indicated sources are from relevant literature. The prescriptions without sources indicated are those created by the author.

TIAN DONG BING ZI

Main Ingredients

Tian Dong (Radix asparagi)	500 grams
Bai Mi (Mel)	100 grams
Hu Ma Mo (*Semen sesami* in the form of fine powder)	200 grams
Hei Dou Huang Mo (*Glycine max* seeds in the form of fine powder)	an adequate amount

Preparation

Pound *Tian Dong* to get 150 grams of its juice, and decoct the juice until 50 grams of it remains. Place *Bai Mi* and *Hu Ma Mo*, which has been slightly parched, into the juice and stir the mixture evenly. Add an appropriate amount of *Hei Dou Huang Mo* to the mixture and make the final mixture into pancakes, each of which is 9 cm. in diameter and 15 cm. in thickness. Steam and then bake in a pan or roast the pancakes until they are done.

Dosage and Administration

Take one three times a day. Chew well and swallow with warm liquor.

Effect

Nourishes *yin*-essence, supplements the lungs and kidneys, makes teeth strong and hair dark.

Indications

Impairments due to deficiency, infirmity with age, emaciation, and other disorders due to *yin*-deficiency of the lungs and kidneys.

Notes

Both *Tian Men Dong* and *Hu Ma* are anti-aging agents.

Source

Tai Ping Sheng Hui Fang (*Peaceful Holy Benevolent Prescriptions*)

Main Ingredients

Huang Jing (*Rhizoma polygonati*)	an adequate amount
Hei Dou Huang Mo (*Clycine max* seeds in the form of fine powder)	an adequate amount

Preparation

Decoct *Huang Jing* in water and condense the decoction into a jelly. Mix the jelly with *Hei Dou Huang Mo,* which has been parched, and make the mixture into coin-sized pancakes. Finally steam or bake the pancakes until they are done.

Dosage and Administration

Take two of them daily.

Effect

Invigorates vital essence, benefits bone marrow, nourishes *yin*, replenishes *qi*, and strengthens tendons and bones.

Indications

Lack of vital essence and bone marrow, *qi*-weakness due to deficiency of *yin*, fatigue, inability of the limbs, and hemoptysis due to impairment of the lungs.

Source

Tai Ping Sheng Hui Fang

Main Ingredients

Pao Fu Zi (*Radix aconiti lateralis preparata*)	30 grams
Shen Qu (*Massa fermentata medicinalis*)	90 grams
Pao Gan Jiang (*Rhizoma zingiberis praeparata*)	90 grams
Zao (*Fructus jujubae*)	30 dates
Gui Xin (*Cortex cinnamomi*)	30 grams
Wu Wei Zi (*Fructus schisandrae*)	30 grams
Tu Si Zi (*Semen cuscutae*)	30 grams
Rou Cong Rong (*Herba cistanchis*)	30 grams
Shu Bao (*Pericarpium zanthoxyli*)	15 grams
Yang Sui (sheep marrow)	90 grams
Su (butter)	60 grams
Mi (*Mel*)	120 grams
Huang Yang Ru (milk)	1.5 litres
Bai Mian (flour)	500 grams

Preparation

Peel *Pao Fu Zi.* Remove the skirt and core of *Zao.* Steep *Rou Cong Rong* for one day and night, remove its shrunken skin, and fry it dry. Parch *Shu Jiao* a little until it becomes slightly yellow. Grind the processed *Pao Fu Zi, Tu Si Zi, Rou Cong Rong,* and *Shu Jiao* together with *Shen Qu, Pao Gan Jiang, Gui Xin,* and *Wu Wei Zi* into a fine powder. Mix the powder with *Bai Mian, Su, Yang Sui, Mi* and *Yang Ru* into a mixture, and add *Zao.* Cook the mixture and put it in a basin with a tight cover. Immediately after the basin has been left in a ventilated place for half a day, remove the contents, prepare it, and cook it again. Make the contents into pancakes. Finally roast them in an oven until they are done.

Dosage and Administration

Take one the pancake daily on an empty stomach.

Effect

Warms the kidney-*yang*, dispels *yin*-cold, and supplements vital essence and the marrow.

Indications

Deficiency of the kidney-*yang*, decline of fire in the gate of life, weakness and impairment due to insufficiency of vital essence and marrow, impotence, emission, frequent urination at night, lassitude of the loins and knees, aversion to cold, and cold limbs.

Notes

Fu Zi is hot in nature and toxicity. It must be processed before being used, and overuse should be avoided. The pancakes containing it should be small in size and should not be taken in excess amount.

Source

The writing, *Lao Lao Yu Bian*, by Xu Chunfu in the Ming dynasty

QI YI BING

Main Ingredients

Sheng Qian Shi (Semen euryales)	180 grams
Sheng Ji Nei Jin (Endothelium corneum gigeriae galli)	90 grams
Bai Mian (flour)	250 grams
Bai Sha Tang (Sacharum)	an adequate amount

Preparation

First grind *Sheng Qian Shi* and strain the powder. Then grind and strain *Sheng Ji Nei Jin*, and infuse the powder with boiling water. Steep it in water for about a half day. Take out the steeped *Ji Nei Jin* and mix it with the fine powders of *Qian Shi*, *Bai Mian* and *Bai Sha Tang*. Make the mixture into pancakes with the water in which *Ji Nei Jin* has been steeped. Finally bake the pancakes in a pan until they become yellowish.

Dosage and Administration

Eat freely.

Effect

Strengthens the kidneys, stops nocturnal emissions, and invigorates the spleen to promote digestion.

Indications

Deficiency of *qi* indicated by failure to cough up sputum, retention of phlegm, stagnation of *qi*, fullness in the chest, hypochondriac pain, and hernia.

These pancakes are effective for those that are ill with the syndrome of deficiency of vital energy and cough-producing sputum.

Source
Yi Xue Zhong Zhong Can Xi Lu

Main Ingredients

Bai Zhu (Rhizoma atractylodis macrocephalae)	120 grams
Ji Nei Jin (Endothehum corneum gigeriae galli)	60 grams
Gan Jiang (Rhizoma zingiberis)	60 grams
Shu Zao Rou (Fructus jujubae)	250 grams

Preparation
Grind *Bai Zhu* into powder and bake the powder until it is done. Do the same with *Ji Nei Jin*. Smash *Gan Jiang* and pound all the above into a paste. Make the paste into small pancakes. Finally fry the pancakes to dry them.

Dosage and Administration
Pancakes of this kind are to be eaten as a snack. Chew well.

Effect
Strengthens the spleen, warms the stomach, replenishes *qi*, nourishes blood, and promotes digestion.

Indications
Syndrome due to weakness of the spleen and stomach accompanied by cold, pain in the hypochondriac and abdominal region, frequent and sudden diarrhea, indigestion that is aggravated by cold or fatigue.

Source
Yi Xue Zhong Zhong Can Xi Lu

Main Ingredients

Fu Ling (Poria)	30 grams
Shan Yao (Rhizoma dioscoreae)	30 grams
He Shou Wu (Radix polygoni multiflori)	30 grams
Lian Zi Rou (Semen nelumbinis)	30 grams
Gou Qi Zi (Fructus lycii)	30 grams
Bai Mian (flour)	500 grams
Bai Tang (Sacharum)	an adequate amount

Preparation
Grind the first five ingredients into fine powder. Mix the powder, *Bai Mian*, and *Bai Tang* evenly with water into a paste. Make the paste into pancakes, and bake the pancakes in the form of a biscuit.

Dosage and Administration
The pancakes are for one-week use.

Effect

Invigorates both the spleen and the kidneys and supplements *qi* and vital essence.

Indications

Early senility, weakness of the body, and deficiency of both the spleen and the kidneys.

JIU XIAN BAO JIAN BING

Main Ingredients

Fu Ling (Poria)	30 grams
Shan Yao (Rhizoma dioscoreae)	30 grams
Yi Mi (Semen Coicis)	30 grams
Qian Shi (Semen eutyales)	30 grams
Bai He (Bulbus lilii)	30 grams
Chao Shan Zha (parched *Fructus grataegi*)	30 grams
Chao Mai Ya (parched *Fructus hordei germinatus*)	30 grams
Sha Ren (Fructus amomi)	9 grams
Chao Hei Zhi Ma (Semen sesami nigrum)	30 grams
Mian Fen (flour)	100 grams
Bai Tang (white sugar)	an adequate amount

Preparation

Grind the first eight ingredients into fine powder. Mix the powder with *Chao Hei Zhi Ma* and *Bai Tang* into an even mixture. Mix with water into a dough. Form the dough into small pancakes like biscuits. Bake or roast the pancakes until they are done.

Dosage and Administration

Eat at will.

Effect

Replenishes the heart and spleen, tonifies the liver and kidneys, stops nocturnal emissions, calms the mind, nourishes the five *zang* organs, strengthens the stomach, activates the flow of *qi*, and promotes digestion.

CHAPTER 3

Healthcare Independent of Medicines

3.1 Acupuncture and Moxibustion for Healthcare

Acupuncture and moxibustion are healthcare practices that are unique to the Chinese nation. They have made great contributions to the healthcare profession in general, and today such practices are well accepted and highly appreciated throughout the world.

Acupuncturology involves two therapies: acupuncture and moxibustion. These therapies were formed and developed gradually in the struggle of human beings against diseases. As early as 10,000 years ago, the Chinese already knew that puncturing some parts of the body with chipped stone instruments could alleviate the sufferings due to disorders. This was the beginning of acupuncture. Up to the New Stone Age, the Chinese people used polished stone needles as special medical instruments, which were then called *Bian Shi*. Later on, with the development of social productive forces, science, and technology, the Chinese continued to improve acupuncture instruments making them from bamboo and then bone.

Throughout history, the needles were continually improved upon as they were made of bronze, iron, gold, silver and stainless steel. As fire came into use, it was found out that the sufferings due to disease could be relieved when some parts of the body were heated. This was the beginning of combustion therapy, which was later developed into moxibustion and other kinds of combustion therapies. The ancient Chinese people summarized their rich practical experiences with acupuncture and moxibustion in a whole series of integrated scientific theories. In recent years, modern scientific research in acupuncture and moxibustion has been carried out both theoretically and clinically, resulting in a more rapid development of this science.

Both acupuncture and moxibustion can be used to promote health and prevent diseases.

3.1.1 THE EFFECTS OF ACUPUNCTURE AND MOXIBUSTION IN HEALTHCARE

When you are healthy, the *yin* and *yang* in your body are in harmony, *qi* and blood exuberate, *zang* and *fu* function well, the channels and collaterals are smooth, and *ying* and *wei* harmonize. When you are not healthy, the conditions are just the opposite. Acupuncture and moxibustion act on the acupoints, channels, and collaterals to clear them and, thus, promote the flow of *qi* and blood, harmonize *yin* and *yang*, regulate *zang* and *fu*, harmonize *ying* and *wei*, eliminate diseases, and expel pathogenic factors. These regulating effects of acupuncture and moxibustion can, of course, ensure perfect health, prevent early aging, and prolong life.

Actions of Moxibustion

Warming and Clearing Channels and Collaterals to Remove *Yin*-cold. Moxibustion is a kind of warm stimulation that disperses cold pathogens. It can be used to warm and clear the channels, collaterals, and blood vessels, expel wind-dampness, and *yin*-pathogens of wind-cold type. It also prevents the invasion of wind, cold, and damp pathogens and is used to treat and prevent arthritis.

Supplementing Fire and Strengthening *Yang* to Retard Senility. Moxibustion treatments on the acupoints *Shenque* (RN8), *Guanyuan* (RN4), *Qihai* (RN6), *Mingmen* (DU4) and *Shenshu* (BL23) can enhance vitality and slow down the process of aging. The heat given off by the moxa burning over the acupoints, in combination with its warm nature and fragrance, strengthens the fire from the gate of life and warms and reinforces *yang-qi*.

Supporting Vital-*qi* to Prevent Diseases. It is very hard for the weak or the old to guard themselves against the invasion of exogenous pathogens because they have deficient vital-*qi*, weakened *zang* and *fu*, and loose striae. Therefore, the six evils may take the opportunity to break through their body's defenses, causing them to be ill or even die. Moxibustion for healthcare can be used, in this case, to support vital-*qi*, supplement primordial-*qi*, close the striae of the skin properly, and improve the functions of *zang* and *fu* organs, thus strengthening their ability to prevent disease. People who are susceptible to diseases due to poor health, especially those over middle age, should be treated with moxibustion.

Invigorating the Spleen and Stomach to Strengthen the Acquired *Qi* after Birth. The spleen and stomach are the material basis of the acquired constitution of the body. If they function normally in receiving, transporting, and digesting food, they will provide the body with enough essential substances to enhance essence and blood and build up health. Regular applications of moxibustion over the acupoints, *Zusanli* (ST36) and *Zongwan* (RN12), will warm the spleen-*yang*, replenish stomach-*qi*, and promote digestion.

Promoting the Flow of *Qi* and Blood to Resolve Masses and Relieving Swelling. In the healthy body, *qi* and blood move freely. Any stagnation of them will obstruct the channels and collaterals and result in blood-stasis and phlegm-retention. This, in turn, can lead to masses in the abdomen, swelling, and apoplexy. If moxibustion is regularly applied, *qi* and blood will be kept flowing and the channels and collaterals will remain clear and smooth, which will prevent the above mentioned syndromes.

3.1.2 MECHANISMS OF ACUPUNCTURE AND MOXIBUSTION

The following are mechanisms that modern research has proven to be a result of acupuncture and moxibustion.

Improving Immunologic Function. Acupuncture and moxibustion can enhance cellular immune functions. For example, they can regulate the count and the activities of the lymphocytes in peripheral blood, adjust the total number of leucocytes in peripheral blood flow, strengthen the function of the reticuloendothelial system, control the content of immunoglobulin in blood sera, and increase the content of complements in blood sera. Thus, acupuncture and moxibustion can produce the effects of preventing diseases, preserving health, and slowing down the process of aging.

Adjusting Cardiovascular Function to Improve Microcirculation. Acupuncture and moxibustion have good regulative effects on the functions of the heart and blood vessels. For example, they can cause vasoconstriction, adjust blood pressure, and improve the function of the heart, coronary circulation, and microcirculation. For this reason, acupuncture and moxibustion may be used to prevent cardiovascular diseases and promote the recovery of the patients who have been ill with those diseases.

Improving the Function of Digestion and Absorption. Application of acupunction and moxibustion to acupoints such as *Zusanli* (ST36) may attain the effect of regulating gastrointestinal peristalsis to promote the digestion of food and the absorption of nutrients, thus harmonizing the whole digestive system. This can build up constitution and strengthen the resistance to diseases.

Improving the Functions of Many Other Systems. Application of acupuncture and moxibustion can regulate the function of the nervous system and the functions of endocrine glands such as the pituitary and adrenal glands. They can also help the functions of respiration, urination, and reproduction.

3.1.3 COMMONLY SELECTED ACUPOINTS IN HEALTHCARE

The theoretical basis of acupuncture and moxibustion is the theory of the channels and collaterals. Channels and collaterals are the passages through which the *qi* and blood of the body flow. They are everywhere in the body, throughout the *zang-fu* organs, uniting all the tissues and organs into an organic whole. The channel system includes twelve regular channels and eight extra channels.

Acupoints, usually called points for short, are specific locations on (or over) which acupuncture or moxibustion is applied. When these points are stimulated, they will play a part in promoting the flow of *qi* and blood, thus, strengthening the body's resistance to pathogenic factors. The acupoints include 361 points from the fourteen channels (the twelve channels plus *Du* channel and *Ren* channel), extra points, and *Ashi* points. Locating or selecting the acupoints accurately (or not) is closely related to the curative effects of this science. Location of the points is key. The following are three methods for doing so.

Gu Du Fen Cun Ce Liang Fa

The *Cun* is a unit used for measuring different parts of the body. For example the measurement of the length from the center of the navel up to the juncture between pectus major and xiphoid process is equal to 8 *Cun*. That distance down to the upper border of the symphysis pubis is equal to 5 *Cun*. The length of the *Cun* is used to locate points.

Shou Zhi Tong Shen Cun Fa

In this method, the lengths of patient's fingers are regarded as *Cun*. There are three kinds of this type of *Cun*.

1. ***Zhong Zhi Tong Shen Cun.*** The length between the first and second knuckles in the inner lateral side of the middle finger when it is bent is regarded as one *Cun*.

2. ***Mu Zhi Tong Shen Cun.*** The width of the knuckle of the thumb of the patient is regarded as one *Cun*.

3. ***Heng Zhi Tong Shen Cun.*** The width of the four fingers of a patient measured at the second knuckle of the middle finger is regarded as 3 *Cun*.

Ti Biao Biao Zhi Fa

Anatomic marks of the body, fixed, or as they appear when the body is in a certain posture, are also regarded as the basis of point selection.

The following is a description of the locations of the more commonly selected healthcare points. For details of all the other points, channels, and collaterals, please consult relevant works on acumoxibustion.

ZUSANLI (ST36)

Location

3 *Cun* directly below *Dubi* (ST35), one finger-breadth from the anterior crest of the tibia or in the anterior tibia muscle.

Method

Puncture perpendicularly 0.5–1.2 *Cun*. Moxibustion is applicable.

Effect

Regular application of acupuncture and moxibustion on this point will strengthen the function of the spleen and stomach, build up the body, and enhance immunity to disease.

Indications

Disorders of the spleen, stomach, kidneys, liver, heart, lungs, and brain. Indications also include stomachache, vomiting, hiccups, abdominal distension, diarrhea, dysentery, constipation, acute appendicitis, indigestion, apoplexy, paralysis, dizziness, insomnia, mania, cough, edema, acute mastitis, beriberi, soreness of the knees and calves, emaciation due to consumption, and infantile malnutrition.

Notes

This is an essential point commonly chosen for healthcare. Legend has it that there was an old man who had moxibustion done on the *Zusanli* point once daily in the first eight days of each month. He ensured a life span of more than 174 years.

SHENQUE (RN8)

Location

At the center of the umbilicus.

Method

Puncture is prohibited. Moxibustion is applicable.

Effect

Application of moxibustion on this point will reinforce *yang*, supplement *qi*, warm the kidneys, and strengthen the function of the spleen.

Indications

Abdominal pain, flaccidity, apoplexy, and prolapse of the rectum.

Notes

For healthcare, moxibustion is regularly applied on this point.

It is recorded in medical literature that there was an old man who had moxibustion done on the *Shenque* point every year and still kept fit at the age of over 100 years old.

ZHONGJI (RN3)

Location
4 *Cun* below the centre of the umbilicus.
Method
Puncture perpendicularly 0.5–1.0 *Cun*. Moxibustion is applicable.
Indications
Impotence, enuresis, nocturnal emission, frequent urination, retention of urine, metrorrhagia and metrostaxis, irregular menstruation, dysmenorrhea, morbid leukorrhea, pruritus vulvae, prolapse of uterus, pain in the lower abdomen, and hernia.

GUANYUAN (RN4)

Location
3 *Cun* below the center of the umbilicus.
Method
Puncture perpendicularly 0.8–1.2 *Cun*. Moxibustion is applicable.
Indications
Impotence, enuresis, nocturnal emission, frequent urination, retention of urine, uterine bleeding, irregular menstruation, dysmenorrhea, morbid leukorrhea, postpartum hemorrhage, lower abdominal pain, hernia, indigestion, diarrhea, and prolapse of the rectum.
Notes
This is an essential point for building up health.

QIHAI (RN6)

Location
1.5 *Cun* below the centre of the umbilicus.
Method
Puncture perpendicularly 0.8–1.2 *Cun*. Moxibustion is applicable.
Effect
Supplements the kidneys, supports *yang*, replenishes *qi*, and controls nocturnal emissions.
Indications
Impotence, enuresis, nocturnal emission, uterine bleeding, irregular menstruation, dysmenorrhea, amenorrhea, morbid leukorrhea, postpartum hemorrhage, abdominal pain, hernia, diarrhea, dysentery, constipation, edema, flaccid type of apoplexy, and dyspnea.

Notes
This is an essential point for strengthening the body and preserving health.

SHENSHU (BL 23)

Location
On the low back, below the spinous process of the 2nd lumbar vertebra and 1.5 *Cun* lateral to the posterior midline.
Method
Puncture perpendicularly 0.8–1.2 *Cun*. Moxibustion is applicable.
Effect
Tonifies the kidneys, strengthens *yang*, and replenishes vital essence.
Indications
Impotence, nocturnal emission, enuresis, irregular menstruation, morbid leukorrhea, lumbar pain, weakness of the loins and knees, dizziness, tinnitus, deafness, edema, dyspnea, and diarrhea.

MINGMEN (DU 4)

Location
Located on the low back on the posterior midline and in the depression below the spinous process of the 2nd lumbar vertebra.
Method
Puncture perpendicularly 0.5–1.0 *Cun*. Moxibustion is applicable.
Effect
Tonifies the kidneys, strengthens *yang*, and reinforces the stomach.
Indications
Stiffness of the back, lumbago, impotence, nocturnal emission, irregular menstruation, morbid leukorrhea, diarrhea, indigestion, edema, dizziness, and tinnitus.

SANYINJIAO (SP 6)

Location
Posterior to the medial border of the tibia and 3 *Cun* above the tip of the medial malleolus.
Method
Puncture perpendicularly 0.5–1.0 *Cun*. Moxibustion is applicable. Acupuncture on this point is not to be performed on pregnant women.
Indications
Impotence, nocturnal emission, enuresis, uterine bleeding,

irregular menstruation, dysmenorrhea, morbid leukorrhea, abdominal distension, diarrhea, edema, hernia, pain in the external genitalia, paralysis and pain of the lower extremities, headache, dizziness, and insomnia.

ZHONGWAN (RN12)

Location

3 *cun* or 4 *Cun* below the xiphoid process (on the midline of the abdomen) and 4 *Cun* above the umbilicus.

Method

Puncture perpendicularly 0.5–1.2 *Cun*. Moxibustion is applicable.

Indications

Stomachache, acid regurgitation, regurgitation of food from the stomach, vomiting, indigestion, diarrhea, dysentery, jaundice, and insomnia.

Notes

Regular application of moxibustion on this point and *Zusanli* can strengthen the spleen and stomach, and build up the body's constitution.

TIANSHU (ST 25)

Location

In the depression, 2 *Cun* lateral to the centre of the umbilicus.

Method

Puncture perpendicularly 1.0–1.5 *Cun*. Moxibustion is applicable.

Indications

All diseases of the digestive system such as abdominal pain and distension, pain around the umbilicus, diarrhea, dysentery, and constipation, as well as irregular menstruation and edema.

QUCHI (LI 11)

Location

Located on the lateral end of the cubital crease and at the midpoint of the line connecting *Chize* (LU5) and the external humeral epicondyle, when the elbow is flexed.

Method

Puncture perpendicularly 1.0–1.5 *Cun*. Moxibustion is applicable.

Indications

Sore throat, toothache, redness and pain of the eye, scrofula, urticaria, motor impairment of the upper extremities, abdominal pain, vomiting, diarrhea, and febrile disease.

Notes

Regular application of moxibustion on this point and *Zusanli* can regulate blood pressure, prevent apoplexy and enhance resistance to disease.

NEIGUAN (PC6)

Location

Located on the palmar side of the forearm on the line connecting *Quze* (PC3) and *Daling* (PC7), 2 *Cun* above the crease of the wrist between the tendons of the long palmar muscle and radial flexor muscle of the wrist.

Method

Puncture perpendicularly 0.5–0.8 *Cun*. Moxibustion is applicable.

Effect

Regulates effectively the cardiovascular system and preserves health.

Indications

Cardiac pain, palpitations, stuffy chest, mania, epilepsy, insomnia, pain in the hypochondriac region, stomachache, nausea, vomiting, hiccups, febrile disease, irritability, malaria, and pain of the elbow and arm.

SHENMEN (HI 7)

Location

Located at the ulnar end of the crease of the wrist and in the depression on the radial side of the tendon of the ulnar flexor muscle of the wrist.

Method

Puncture perpendicularly 0.3–0.5 *Cun*. Moxibustion is applicable.

Indications

Cardiac pain, irritability, palpitation, hysteria, amnesia, insomnia, mania, epilepsy, dementia, pain in the hypochondriac region, and yellowish sclera.

DAZHUI (GB 14)

Location

Located below the spinous process of the 7th cervical vertebra, approximately at the level of the shoulders.

Method

Puncture obliquely upward 0.5–1.0 *Cun*. Moxibustion is applicable.

Effect

This is a main point for regulating all the *yang* channels. Acupuncture and moxibustion on this point can support *yang* and regulate the *qi* in the channels and collaterals.

Indications
Neck pain and rigidity, malaria, febrile disease, epilepsy, afternoon fever, cough, dyspnea, common cold, and back stiffness.

FEISHU (BL 13)

Location
Located on the back below the spinous process of the 3rd thoracic vertebra and 1.5 *Cun* lateral to the posterior midline.
Method
Puncture obliquely 0.5–0.7 *Cun*. Moxibustion is applicable.
Indications
Cough, dyspnea, fullness in the chest, chest pain, spitting of blood, afternoon fever, and night sweating.
Notes
Regular moxibustion on the above two points can replenish *qi*, support *yang*, reinforce the lungs, consolidate the superficial resistance, and enhance resistance to exogenous evils, which is especially beneficial to those who are susceptible to the common cold because of their weak constitutions.

XINSHU (BL 15)

Location
Located on the back below the spinous process of the 5th thoracic vertebra and 1.5 *Cun* lateral to the posterior midline.
Method
Puncture obliquely 0.5–0.7 *Cun*. Moxibustion is applicable.
Indications
Cardiac pain, amnesia, palpitations, irritability, mania, epilepsy, cough, spitting of blood, nocturnal emission, and night sweating.
Notes
Acupuncture and moxibustion on this point benefits the heart and lungs.

GANSHU (BL 18)

Location
Located on the back below the spinous process of the 9th thoracic vertebra and 1.5 *Cun* lateral to the posterior midline.
Method
Puncture obliquely 0.5–0.7 *Cun*. Moxibustion is applicable.
Indications
Pain in the hypochondriac region, jaundice, redress of the eye, blurred vision, night blindness, mania, epilepsy, backache, and spitting of blood.

Notes

Acupuncture and moxibustion on this point benefits the liver and gallbladder.

PISHU (BL 20)

Location

Located on the back below the spinous process of the 11th thoracic vertebra and 1.5 *Cun* lateral to the posterior midline.

Method

Puncture obliquely 0.5–0.7 *Cun.* Moxibustion is applicable.

Indications

Epigastric pain, abdominal distension, anorexia, vomiting, diarrhea, dysentery, bloody stools, jaundice, profuse menstruation, edema, and backache.

WEISHU (BL 21)

Location

Located on the back below the spinous process of the 12th thoracic vertebra and 1.5 *Cun* lateral to the posterior midline.

Method

Puncture obliquely 0.5–0.7 *Cun.* Moxibustion is applicable.

Indications

Epigastric pain, anorexia, abdominal distension, regurgitation of food from the stomach, vomiting, diarrhea, and pain in the hypochondriac region.

Notes

Acupuncture and moxibustion on the above two points benefits the spleen and stomach.

HUANTIAO (GB 30)

Location

When the patient lies on his side with the hip flexed, *Huantiao* is located on the lateral side of the thigh at the middle third and lateral third of the line connecting the prominence of the great trochanter and the sacral hiatus.

Method

Puncture perpendicularly 1.5–2.5 *Cun.* Moxibustion is applicable.

Indications

Pain of the lumbar region and thigh, muscular atrophy of the lower limbs, and herniplegia.

YONGQUAN (KI 1)

Location

Located on the sole in the depression appearing on the anterior part of the sole when the foot is in plantar flexion, approximately at the junction of the anterior third and the posterior two thirds of the line connecting the base of the 2nd and 3rd toes and the heel.

Method

Puncture perpendicularly 0.3–0.5 *Cun*. Moxibustion is applicable.

Indications

Headache, dizziness, blurred vision, sore throat, dryness of the tongue, loss of voice, constipation, infantile convulsions, loss of consciousness, and feverish sensation in the sole.

Notes

Regular moxibustion on this point may reinforce the kidney-*yang* and strengthen the body.

BAIHUI (DU 20)

Location

4.5 *Cun* directly above the midpoint of the anterior hairline.

Method

Puncture subcutaneously 0.3–0.5 *Cun*. Moxibustion is applicable.

Indications

Headache, vertigo, tinnitus, nasal obstruction, coma, aphasia by apoplexy, mania, and prolapse of the rectum and uterus.

DANZHONG (RN 17)

Location

Located on the anterior midline on the level of the 4th intercostal space and at the midpoint of a line connecting both nipples.

Method

Puncture subcutaneously 0.3–0.5 *Cun*. Moxibustion is applicable.

Indications

Pain and fullness in the chest, cardiac pain, palpitations, dyspnea, hiccups, difficulty in swallowing, and insufficient lactation.

3.1.4 ACUPUNCTURE AND MOXIBUSTION FOR HEALTHCARE

Acupuncture for Healthcare

Filiform Needle Puncturing. Needles with loose handles or hooked tips are not to be used. The needles should be straight, smooth, tough and elastic. Before application, choose a suitable posture for the patient and strictly disinfect the needles and the located points.

There is a variety of acupuncture manipulations, which include *Zhiqie* Insertion, *Pianzhi* Insertion, *Shuzhang* Insertion, and *Jiachi* Insertion. It is important that while a needle is being inserted, its angle and depth should be properly controlled. After the insertion, a certain kind of needle transmission is needed to a certain a degree so that the stimulation induced in this way may be felt by the patient. When the patient has a sense of numbness, distention, and compression, the acupuncturist must also have in his finger a sense of sinking and tension. This is called *Deqi*, a state in which the therapeutic efficacy has been achieved. Only when this state appears can a satisfactory curative effect be obtained. After *Deqi*, the needle is generally retained for 15–20 minutes, during which the needle may be manipulated intermittently, keeping or enhancing the stimulation.

When withdrawing the needle, press the skin around the point with the thumb and forefinger of the left hand and twist the needle slowly first to the subcutaneous layer and then out with the right hand. Press the point with a disinfected cotton ball to prevent bleeding.

Cutaneous Needle Puncturing. Plum-blossom needles and seven-star needles are both called cutaneous needles. They are used to tap on the skin the points and the superficial meridians so as to promote *qi* and blood flow through the meridians and to regulate the functions of *zang* and *fu* organs.

A seven-star needle has a handle 17–20 cm. long and a tiny plate in the shape of a lotus seedpod at one end. On the "seedpod," are seven short pins made of stainless steel.

A plum-blossom needle has a handle about 33 cm. long and five to seven stainless steel pins bound tightly together at one end.

The tips of these two kinds of needles must be neither too sharp nor hooked.

In the course of acupuncture, the acupuncturist should strictly disinfect the needle and the skin around the located points, hold the back end of the handle and jerk the wrist quickly to let the other end of the needle quickly tap vertically down and up on the skin. Tap either slightly until the skin becomes congested or until bleeding is about to appear. Finally disinfect the skin.

The location which cutaneous needles are used to tap is usually the route along which the relevant meridian goes and the related points are distributed. For building up constitution, the following points are often chosen: the midline of the back and waist (*Du* Channel) and the four channels (Urinary Bladder Channel of Foot-*Taiyang*), two at the either side: one 1.5 *Cun* and the other 3 *Cun* away from the midline.

Cutaneous needle puncturing is also administered to prevent and treat headache, dizziness, insomnia, gastrointestinal diseases, women's diseases, cutaneous diseases, flaccidity, and arthralgia syndromes.

Intradermal Needle Puncturing. Intradermal needles are usually made of 30–32 sizes of stainless steel wire and are short. They come in two shapes: thumbtack-shaped and wheatgrain-shaped. The former is about 0.3 cm. long and used mainly on the auricles while the latter is 1 cm. long and is used on acupoints or pressure pain points all over the body.

In application, the needles are buried under the skin. This kind of puncturing is also called needle-embedding therapy. Because the needles buried under the skin are always retained for a certain time, continuous stimulation is then achieved. This meets the purpose of healthcare and the treatment of various chronic and ache-causing diseases among which are headache, stomachache, insomnia, asthma, enuresis, dysmenorrhea, and some menstrual disturbances.

The method of operation is as follows: Disinfect the needle and the area thoroughly.

Insert the needle with a pair of sterilized tweezers into the skin with its handle remaining outside. Fix it with a piece of adhesive plaster. In summer, the needle is not to be retained for more than two days lest infection occur but in winter or autumn, it can be left in longer if necessary. Needle-embedding near the joints and on the purulent skin is not allowed.

Moxibustion for Healthcare

Moxibustion consists of the following three kinds: moxa cone moxibustion, moxa roll moxibustion, and needle-warming through moxibustion. As its name indicates, needle-warming though moxibustion is a treatment in which needling and moxibustion are used in combination. It is not introduced here in detail.

Leaves of moxa, belonging to those of the composite family, are warm in nature and fragrant and acrid in flavor. They support *yang-qi*, warm the meridians, expel cold, and dredge the meridian passages to regulate *qi* and blood. To make moxa, Chinese mugwort leaves are pounded into mugwort floss, which is easily lit. When burning, it produces a moderate heat which tends to the skin and enters the muscles.

Moxa cones are made in the following ways. A small amount of mugwort floss is put over a flat surface and molded into circular cones with the thumb, forefinger, and middle finger. The small cones are as big as wheat grains or half the size of date cores and are used in direct moxibustion. The larger ones are as big as thumbs, each about 1 cm. high and with a base whose diameter is 0.8 cm. They are used in indirect moxibustion. Moxa rolls are made by putting mugwort floss on pieces of mulberry paper and rolling the pieces like a cigar. Each is 20 cm. long and with a base whose diameter is 1.5 cm. These rolls are easy to use in moxa roll moxibustion.

Moxa Cone Moxibustion. There are two ways to perform cone moxibustion: direct and indirect. When you burn one cone up it is known as one *Zhuang*.

Direct moxibustion is performed by placing a moxa cone directly on an acupoint and lighting it. This method was popular in ancient times. There are two types of direct moxibustion: non-scarring and scarring. Non-scarring moxibustion is performed by allowing the cone to burn only half way down so that the skin does not burn or blister. Scarring moxibustion on the other hand is rarely practiced any more because of the pain involved and the damage that it does to the skin. When scarring moxibustion was practiced, scallion or garlic juice was first applied to the point. Then the cone was applied and lit and allowed to burn down. This would cause the skin to burn, blister, and fester following the treatment.

Indirect moxibustion is also called indirect contact moxibustion. It is applied by placing adequate medicines between the skin and the moxa cone, preventing the skin from being directly burned and bringing the medicines' effects into play. Indirect moxibustion varies according to the different medicines used. For example, there is ginger moxibustion, garlic moxibustion, moxibustion with salt, and moxibustion with *Fu Zi Bing*, each being used to treat a different ailment. Ginger moxibustion is used to treat the syndrome due to *yang*-deficiency, such as weakness of the spleen and stomach, diarrhea, abdominal pain and stagnation of *qi*. Garlic moxibustion is used to treat insect-bites and skin and external diseases that are in early stages. Moxibustion with *Fu Zi Bing* is used to treat impotence and premature ejaculation due to deficiency of the kidney-*yang*, as well as obstinate syndromes due to *yin*-cold or deficiency. Moxibustion with salt is applied on the acupoint *Shenjue* (RN 8), which helps the recuperation of depleted *yang* and treats abdominal pain, hernia, diarrhea, and long-standing dysentery.

Moxa Roll Moxibustion. Moxa roll moxibustion is commonly used today in healthcare. With this type of indirect moxibustion, the points are selected and then heated with a lit moxa roll. This method consists of mild moxibustion and bird-pecking moxibustion.

Mild Moxibustion. Smoke and heat the points chosen with the lit end of a moxa roll at a certain distance from the skin until the skin feels hot and becomes reddish. This is usually done in intervals of 5–10 minutes.

Bird-pecking Moxibustion. Move the lit end of a moxa roll up and down above the point like a bird pecks grains, or move it evenly from the right to the left (or horizontally) over the point.

SELECTION AND COMPATIBILITY OF POINTS IN ACUPUNCTURE AND MOXIBUSTION FOR HEALTHCARE*

Points Selected for the Purpose of Strengthening Health and Prolonging Life:

- Zusanli (ST 36)
- Shenque (RN 8)
- Guanyuan (RN 4)
- Qihai (RN 6)
- Dazhui (GB 14)
- Yongquan (KI 1)

Points Selected for the Purpose of Invigorating the Kidney-yang to Stop Nocturnal Emission:

- Mingmen (DU 4)
- Shenshu (BL 23)
- Zhongji (RN 3)
- Guanyuan (RN 4)
- Qihai (RN 6)
- SanYinjiao (SP 6)
- Yongquan (KI 1)

Points Selected for the Purpose of Replenishing Qi of the Spleen and Stomach to Strengthen the Digestive System:

- Zusanli (ST 36)
- Zhongwan (RN 12)
- Tianshu (ST 25)
- Pishu (BL 20)
- Weieshu (BL 21)
- Shenque (RN 8)

Points Selected to Keep the Circulatory System Healthy:

- Xinshu (BL 15)
- Neiguan (PC 6)
- Danzhong (RN17)
- Shemnen (HT7)

Points Selected to Keep the Respiratory System Healthy:

- Feishu (BL 13)
- Dazhui (GB 14)
- Xinshu (BL 15)
- Danzhong (RN 17)

Points Selected to Keep the Urinary and Reproductive Systems Healthy:

- Shenshu (BL 23)
- Mingmen (DU 4)
- SanYinjiao (SP 6)
- Zhongji (RN 3)
- Guanyuan (RN 4)
- Qihai (RN 6)

Points Selected for Regulating the Mind:

- Shemnen (HT 7)
- Neiguan (PC 6)
- Xinshu (BL 15)
- SanYinjiao (SP 6)

Points Selected for the Prevention and Recovery of Apoplexy:

- Zusanli (ST 36)
- Quchi (LI 11)
- Baihui (DU 20)
- Huantiao (GB 30)

Points Selected for the Prevention and Recovery of Gallbladder Diseases:

- Ganshu (BL 18)
- Pishu (BL 20)
- Zusanli (ST 36)

Points Selected for the Prevention of Cold:

- Dazhui (GB 14)
- Feishu (BL 13)
- Zusanfi (ST 36)

Points Selected for the Auxiliary Treatment and Recovery of Collapse:

- Shenque (RN 8)
- Guanyuan (RN 4)
- Zhongji (RN 3)

Points Selected for the Prevention and Recovery of Lead Diseases:

- Baihui (DU 20)
- Yongquan (KI 1)

Points Selected for the Prevention and Recovery of Waist and Leg Disorders:

- Shenshu (BL 23)
- Mingnien (DU 4)
- Fluantiao (GB 30)
- SanYinjiao (SP 6)

*It is not necessary to use all the points listed above every time in clinical treatment. One to three points are enough for each practical treatment.

The application of any kind of moxibustion must be adequate in its amount. Therefore, be sure to decide how big the moxa cone should be and how long the moxa roll moxibustion should last according to the constitution, the disease condition, the age of the condition, and the age of the patient. Moxibustion that has been overdone can cause blisters. If this does occur, do not rupture them, rather just let them heal naturally.

Cautions in Acupuncture and Moxibustion for Healthcare.

* Moxibustion is used more frequently than acupuncture, especially for the weak and old.
* Comfortable and durable postures are to be chosen for a subject such as supine and sitting.
* Points in the lower abdominal and lumbosacral areas are not to be used on pregnant women. Special care should be taken to avoid hurting the important internal organs when points on the chest and abdomen are being punctured. It is also extremely important, to be sure all implements and working areas are clean and disinfected.
* When applying moxibustion, be extremely careful not to injure the skin.
* After the application of moxibustion, the subject should not have tea or food immediately. Rather, they should lie down so as not to be bothered by anything.
* Regular application of acupuncture and moxibustion for healthcare is especially important. One course of treatment consists of ten applications.

3.2 *Qigong* Exercises for Healthcare

Qigong is a traditional exercise created by the labor workers of China for keeping fit. It is good for people of all ages, especially for the elderly and middle-aged. *Qigong* includes: *Daoyin* (inducement of *qi* by the mind), *Tuna* (breathing out and in), *Zuochan* (sitting in meditation), *Anqiao* (self-massage at certain acupoints plus *Daoyin* through special posture), and *Jing Zuo* (sitting still, similar to *Zuochan*).

Based on a series of TCM theories with *qi* functioning as the power, *qigong* can help an exerciser achieve self-control, self-adjustment, self-repair, and self-building, as well as enable him or her to prevent and combat diseases and preserve good health.

The basic patterns of *qigong* were formed during the periods of the Spring-Autumn and Warring States and have been continuously been developed ever since. Through the centuries, many different schools of *qigong* have been formed because of different views of the theory and different ways of exercising. There are, for example, dynamic *qigong*, static *qigong*, health-preserving, hard *qigong*, pneumatic *Neigong*, and vocal *qigong*. Additionally, there is *qigong* for building up health, *qigong* for treating diseases, internal *qigong* and out-going-*qi qigong* (to name but a few). Though the ways of exercising of a particular school may differ, the fundamental principles remain the same.

All schools emphasize a way of exercising that is used to improve *jing* (essence), *qi* (vital energy) and *shen* (vitality) as well as to toughen *jin* (muscles and tendons), *gu* (bones) and *pi* (skin). By practicing *qigong* exercises, the exerciser can maintain a sound mind, regulate *qi* and blood, establish good balance between *yin* and *yang*, and activate blood circulation to remove blood stasis, which will make it possible for him or her to prevent and combat diseases and ensure a long life.

Included in this section is but a brief introduction to ways of exercising and schools of *qigong* exercises. For detailed information, please refer to related treatises on *qigong*.

3.2.1 WAYS OF EXERCISING

Ways of exercising refer to ways in doing *qigong* exercises. Because there are so many different ways of doing this, it is necessary to summarize them. In a word, practicing *qigong* exercises means to train oneself both mentally and physically by giving full play to one's subjective initiative to reach the goal of preserving good health and overcoming diseases.

Qigong exercises, whatever school they may pertain to, include Three Regulations that associate, influence, and promote each other. They are: the regulation of posture, the regulation of mental activities, and the regulation of respiration.

Regulation of Posture

Regulation of posture refers to choosing a specific posture when doing exercises. There are normally four basic postures, which include standing, sitting, lying down, and walking. As a general rule, sitting is the most frequently selected posture in practice.

Standing Posture. This posture is usually used to build up a strong constitution. The following explains how to practice the standing posture.

- Stand with the feet shoulder-width apart. Allow the knee joints to flex a little and the toes to point slightly inward.
- Withdraw the chest properly.
- Raise the arms first to the level of the shoulders and then let

them down slowly with the hands about 30 cm. apart at the height of the nipples.

- Keep this posture as if you were holding a ball.
- Narrow your eyes and mouth, and smile.

Sitting Posture. The more commonly selected modes include sitting upright on a stool, sitting crossed-legged freely on a board bed, and sitting on a board bed with one sole upward.

- Sitting Upright. Sit upright on a stool with your feet on the ground, and your legs apart from each other. A right angle must be formed between the body trunk and the legs and between the thighs and the calves. Place your hands in fists on your knees or in front of your lower abdomen. Tuck your chin, relax your shoulders, and hollow your chest. Narrow your eyes and mouth, and place your tongue to your palate and smile softly.

- Sitting Cross-legged Freely. This posture requires the exerciser is to sit upright cross-legged (knees outward and soles inward) on a hard board. The other principles are the same as those mentioned above.

- Sitting Cross-legged with One Sole Upward. This mode also requires the exerciser to sit upright cross-legged on a hard board, but he or she needs to do this with the knees outward and either of the soles upward crossing the calf of the other leg. The rest of the requirements are the same as those in the first mode.

Lying Posture. This posture preferred by patients who are weak due to prolonged illness or by patients who suffer from insufficiency of *yang-qi* or other chronic diseases. This posture has two modes.

- Lying in Dorsal Position. This mode requires the exerciser to lie dorsally on hard board, while the upper part of the body is raised to an oblique position. The legs should be stretched straight, and the hands are at rest at either side of the body. Narrowed eyes and mouth and a smile are also required.

- Lying in Lateral Recumbent Position. This mode requires the exerciser to lie on one's side hard with the head resting on a pillow and kept at the same level as the body. The upper part of the body should be kept straight with one leg flexed and riding on the other which is extended. The upper hand is placed against the hip while the lower hand on the pillow with the palm upward. The requirements for narrowed eyes and mouth and a smile are the same as in the posture of sitting upright. It makes no difference on which side you lie; however, patients with heart trouble are advised to lie on their right side.

Walking Manner. This posture is used in both *qigong* exercises and *wushu* (martial arts). Activities vary with schools, but the following is a basic method.

- Stand still for 2–3 minutes before walking.
- Step a pace forward with the left foot. Be sure that the heel touches the ground first while the upper part of the body and the hands swing to the right. Inhale through the nose and exhale through the mouth.
- Take the second step with the right foot and repeat the other movements described above except that the swinging is towards the left.
- Repeat the steps in above alternately for about 20–30 minutes.

Regulation of Mental Activities

Regulation of mental activities is a method by which the exerciser can regulate his or her physiological functions through training of the mind. In doing *qigong* exercises, one can regulate mental activities to reach the state of *rujing*. The level of *rujing* attained determines the result the exerciser can achieve. The better the state is, the greater the result will be. The meaning of *rujing* here is the stable state of stillness that the exerciser can achieve resulting from his or her concentration of the mind on a single part of the body. When the exerciser is in this state, he or she is practically insensitive to external stimulation such as sound and light. Usually, there are five methods to reach the state of *rujing*.

Method of Concentration. This method requires the exerciser to concentrate the mind highly on a certain point of the body. The frequently selected point is *Dantian* or *Qihai* (RN 6). When concentrating the mind on the selected point, the exerciser should expel all distracting thoughts. The best way to perform concentration is to do it naturally and relaxed.

Method of Attention to Respiration. In practicing this method, the exerciser must concentrate the mind on breathing. They must pay attention to the process of inhaling and exhaling of abdominal respiration. To reach the state *rujing*, a harmonious relationship between mind concentration and natural process of breathing should be established.

Method of Counting Breathing. By counting the inhalations and exhalations the exerciser will be able to block out external stimuli and clear the mind.

Method of Recitation in Mind. Before starting the exerciser will select some simple and positive words or expressions that are short and easy to recite. When doing the *qigong* exercises, the exerciser concentrates his or her attention to nothing except reciting these simple words again and again. In doing so the exerciser has already expelled all distracting thoughts from the mind, which will help him or her reach the state of *rujing*.

Method of Listening to Breathing. To follow this method, the exerciser should try to listen to his or her own breathing.

For beginners, it is recommended to choose the Method of Concentration at first. They can gradually practice the other methods, and choose the one that they like best.

Regulation of Respiration

Regulation of respiration is also known as deep respiration or training of breathing. It is one of the most important steps in *qigong* exercises. Regulation here means to change the usual thoracic respiration to abdominal respiration; that is, change shallow breathing into deep breathing through exercises to establish spontaneous *Dantian* respiration. This type of respiration also massages the internal organs to help digestion and absorption. There are eight commonly employed methods of breathing.

Natural Breathing. Natural breathing is also known as physiological respiration. When practicing this type of breathing, the exerciser respires naturally without any interference by the mind. The process of breathing is even and mild although not deep and prolonged.

***Shun* Breathing (breathing with diaphragm-down inhaling).** During this breathing process, the diaphragm moves down and the abdomen expands when the exerciser inhales, and when he or she exhales, the diaphragm moves up and the belly contracts in. This type of breathing enables the diaphragm to move up and down.

***Ni* Breathing (breathing with diaphragm-up inhaling).** This type of breathing may be regarded as the counter-type of *Shun* Breathing. During this process the diaphragm moves up when the exerciser inhales and down when he she exhales. Correspondingly, breathing in makes the abdomen contract and breathing out makes it expand. This type of breathing requires a greater amount of exercise and more strength than *Shun* breathing.

***Tinbi* Breathing (Breathing with prolonged inhalation or exhalation).** This method needs prolonged inhalation and exhalation for one respiration.

Breathing with Nasal Inhalation and Oral Exhalation. This type of breathing is particularly applicable for patients ill with diseases of the respiratory tract that have narrowed the air passage and caused unsmooth respiration. A person practicing this type of respiration, inhales through the nose and exhales through the mouth.

Breathing with *Qi* Travelling through the *Ren* and *Du* Channels. This type of breathing begins with *Ni* breathing. The exerciser breathes in air by the nose and imagines that it is led by the mind down to *Dantian* and further down to the perineum. When the exerciser exhales, the air travels from the perineum through the spine to the point *Baihui* (DU20) and then is breathed out through the nose. As the air circulates vertically once within the body, it is also called *Xiao Zhoutian* breathing or small circle of the evolution.

***Qian* Breathing (sub-breathing).** This is a type of breathing naturally formed after having exercised *Shun* breathing or *Ni* breathing for a period of time. This type of breathing is characterized by extremely mild and considerably prolonged inhalation and a faint exhalation. During this process, the breathing is extremely even. It is called sub-breathing because you can hardly perceive the air current even if you put a finger directly under the nose to test it.

Essential Breathing (very mild abdominal breathing). During this state of breathing, visible ordinary breathing ceases and internal essential breathing naturally begins. What is meant here is that ordinary respiration ceases and gentle abdominal breathing begins. This is the breathing that can be done only by those who have reached the high stage in *Qigong* exercises.

Training of respiration must be combined with protection of respiration. No matter what type of breathing is selected for *qigong* exercises, it must be changed into natural breathing when it has been practiced for 10–20 minutes. Otherwise, the respiratory muscles will be exhausted. Only with patient practice can the exerciser gradually learn to make breathing deep, long, gentle, even, and slow. No hasty attempt can be successful.

3.2.2 TYPES OF *QIGONG* EXERCISES

There are many types of *Qigong* exercises. Such types include *Songfing Gong* (exercises for relaxation and stillness), *Neiyang Gong* (exercises for internal adjustment). and *Qianzhuang Gong* (exercises for building up a strong constitution). They are commonly used to preserve good health, prevent diseases, and procure longevity.

This type of exercise stresses relaxation.

Preparations

The place for doing the exercises should be as quiet as possible and be accessible to fresh air. Be sure to wear loose clothing and rest for about 20 minutes before doing the exercises.

Posture

Assume any of the previously described postures. Be sure that once you correctly assume the posture, you narrow your eyes and gaze at the tip of your nose. Slightly open your mouth, and touch the tip of your tongue to your palate.

The Way to Get Relaxed

Once you have assumed your choice of posture, turn your relaxation to your body. Tuck your chin slightly so as to allow your neck to relax and allow your shoulders to drop naturally. Keep your waist straight with your abdomen slightly pulled in and your chest slightly concave. No part of your body should feel any strain.

Breathing

Songjing Gong exercises require *Shun* breathing. When you inhale say "still" to yourself and when you exhale say "relaxed" to yourself. Your breathing should be natural. It should make you comfortable, and your mind should lead the air down to the *Dantian*. Breathing is one of the key aspects in doing *qigong* exercises, so it must be practiced step by step. It is recommended to practice breath training 20–30 minutes at a time.

Sitting Still

This exercise follows breath training. Sitting still requires concentration of the mind on the navel or *Qihai* (RN 6) without any interference of distracting thoughts. However, stillness is a relative concept, and the state of *rujing* varies with individuals. For a beginner, hasty attempt to reach *rujing* with great effort will never help. When necessary, the exerciser can rid himself or herself of all distracting thoughts by concentrating the mind on one positive idea.

Concluding a Time of Exercising

When you have completed this exercise, press the navel with one palm then place the other palm on top. Move both hands in a counterclockwise fashion allowing the circles to get larger each time. Do this 30 times, then reverse directions and allow the circles to get smaller. When you have finished, you can begin other exercises.

Songjing Gong can be practiced by those individuals that are healthy as well as the middle-aged and elderly. It is also recommended for those individuals with chronic cardiovascular, respiratory, or digestive diseases.

NEIYANG GONG

This type of exercise stresses the regulation of respiration. The requirements for preparations, posture, and the way to get relaxed are the same as those in *Songjing Gong*.

Breathing

When practicing *Neiyang Gong* exercise, the exerciser should practice *Tingbi* breathing. The breathing must be deep and long, soft, gentle, even, and smooth. Each breath should be taken completely through the nose, and the mind should lead the air down to the *Dantian*.

When practicing sitting still during *Neiyang Gong*, the exerciser can use one or two methods to regulate respiration. The other requirements for Sitting Still and Concluding Exercises are the same as those in *Songjing Gong*.

Neiyang Gong is particularly preferable for the elderly, the less able-bodied, and patients with chronic diseases of the digestive system.

QIANGZHUANG GONG

Qiangzhuang Gong puts stress on training to reach the state of *rujing*. As a rule, doing this type of exercise on the basis of *Songjing Gong* will be successful. The key to achieve success lies in correct posture, good regulation of respiration, and high concentration of the mind on the *rujing* state. The requirements for preparations, posture, and the way to get relaxed are the same as those in *Songjing Gong*.

Breathing

Generally, *Shun* breathing is more suitable for males whereas *Ni* breathing is more suitable for females. Breathing practice can last 10–20 minutes before normal respiration is restored. Regulation of respiration in *Qiangzhuang Gong* requires that attention be paid to mild natural exhalation rather than to inhalation.

Sitting Still

Because this exercise aims to train one to reach *rujing*, the exerciser may start sitting still directly without performing the breathing exercise. In order to reach the state of *rujing*, the exercisers can employ any of the ways in Regulation of Mental Activities described earlier. The Sitting Still exercise can take 30–40 minutes.

To conclude the exercises, the exerciser may practice the activities described at the conclusion of *Songjing Gong*.

Qiangzhuang Gong is a unique type of exercise effective in building up a strong constitution, maintaining health, preventing diseases, and ensuring longevity. Its curative effects have proved satisfactory in the treatment of such nervous disorders as neurasthenia, neurosis, and vegetative functional disturbances.

3.2.3 Principles in Doing Qigong Exercises

For the best results, one must possess and practice a good foundation of the following principles:

- When practicing the exercises, you must be confident, resolute, and persistent. You must firmly believe that the exercises are effective in the prevention and treatment of diseases, in keeping fit, and in ensuring longevity.

- Try to avoid any interference from pathogenic emotions and keep yourself in good humor. You should also try to avoid such practices such as smoking and drinking.

- Before beginning exercise, change into loose fitting clothes. It is also important to relax completely and to defecate and urinate if necessary before starting.

- Be sure to choose postures that are most suitable to your constitution and to choose a place that has a good fresh air supply.

- Be sure to warm up and cool down properly.

- Do not fixate on any spontaneous responses that might occur when you are practicing. If something occurs allow it to happen and then let it go.

3.3 TCM Massage for Healthcare

TCM massage is also known as *tuina*. It is an effective therapy that was created by ancestors of the Chinese people through long-term practice and is used to preserve health. TCM massotherapy refers to a method used to treat diseases or to keep good health by applying of continuous skillful actions of the hands or fingers to the skin or muscular tissues of oneself or others. As a treatment, it is economical, safe, effective, easy, and convenient to perform with no need of drugs or medical apparatus. TCM massage is particularly applicable for old people ill with certain chronic diseases.

TCM massage has a long history. It was already in wide medical use in China more than 2,000 years ago, and it has kept developing ever since. Today a complete theoretical system has been formed along with a set of practical and effective manipulative maneuvers.

Because it can cause local or general responses of the body and thus regulate the body's functions and overcome pathogenic factors, TCM massage is used as a therapy to treat diseases and as a method to preserve health. According to TCM theory, massage manipulation applied to the human body may balance *yin* and *yang*, regulate functions, readjust the actions of the meridians, strengthen the body's resistance, eliminate pathogenic factors, promote blood circulation to remove blood stasis, and invigorate the bones and muscles.

The general principle of TCM massotherapy is based on the concept that one must search for the primary cause of diseases in treatment. Choice and performance of manipulative maneuvers depend upon such factors as the patient's age and constitution and the nature and course of the disease.

TCM massage is too broad a text to discuss in this section. We will but concentrate on a brief introduction to self-preservation of health by application of TCM massage. For detailed information, please refer to treatises on *Tuina*.

3.3.1 ACTIVE AND PASSIVE MASSAGE

TCM massage can be classified as active massage and passive massage.

If one performs massage manipulative maneuvers on one's own body to keep in good health, it is termed active massage.

If a doctor performs massage manipulative maneuvers on a patient as a treatment, this is termed passive massage, which is primarily employed to treat diseases.

Difference in performing manipulative maneuvers exists between schools of different views. There are, therefore, various manipulative maneuvers in practicing TCM massage. In general, the following maneuvers can be found in clinical practice:

- Pushing (*Tui*)
- Symmetric pinching (*Na*)
- Pressing (*An*)
- Palm-rubbing (*Mo*)
- Rotatory kneading (*Rou*)
- Mobile finger-pinching (*Nie*)
- Rolling (*Gun*)
- Rubbing (*Ca*)
- Acupoint finger-pushing (*Yun*)
- Foulaging (*Cuo*)
- Holding-and-twisting (*Yao*)
- Rotating (*Nian*)
- Scraping (*Gua*)
- Clapping (*Pai*)

- Piling (*Diè*)
- Fingertip-pressing (*Dian*)
- Pulse-pressing (*Yà*)
- Moderate pulling (*Chen*)
- Finger-flicking (*Tan*)
- Separating (*Fen*)
- Uniting (*Hé*)

The following is a brief description of how to perform the more popular maneuvers.

Pushing Maneuver. Press with a finger, palm, or elbow on a definite part of the patient's body and move it straight and unidirectionally along a certain line for a desired distance. The exertion of strength should be steady and slow, and contact must be maintained. This maneuver can be applied to any part of the body. It increases the excitability of the muscles and promotes blood circulation.

Symmetric Pinching Maneuver. Hold between the fingers and thumb a certain part or point of the patient's body and pinch and release. The performance should be in a moderate and continual way, and any interruption should be avoided. Symmetric pinching can produce such effects as expelling wind and clearing away cold, causing resuscitation and relieving pain, and remitting spasm of the muscles and tendons.

Pressing Maneuver. Press a certain part or acupoint of the patient's body with the fingers or the palm-base and gradually exerts strength downward while rotating. This maneuver has the following modes: thumb-pressing, palm-base pressing, four-finger pressing and two-finger pressing. The pressing can provide a relatively strong stimulation, and it is frequently combined with rotary kneading, forming a compound maneuver known as pressing rotary kneading. Thumb-pressing can be applied to any part of the body; palm-base pressing to the back, waist, and the lower limbs; four-finger pressing to the neck or the costal part; and thumb-and-forefinger-pressing to the fingers or the parts with slim and soft muscles. This maneuver can produce such effects as alleviating pain through inducement, relieving syndromes of stroke, easing constipation, relaxing the muscles, and correcting spinal deformity.

Palm-rubbing Maneuver. Place the palm or the palmar surface of the forefinger, middle finger and ring finger on a certain part of the patient's body and perform rhythmic circular rubbing. When performing this maneuver, be sure that the elbow joint flexes slightly, and that the wrist is relaxed, and that the fingers stretch straight naturally. The rubbing palm or finger surface should move in a circular way under traction of the wrist and forearm. Natural exertion of strength is needed, and the rubbing must be mild and harmonious at a rate of about 120 circles per minute. Palm-rubbing provides mild stimulation and is frequently applied to the thoracic abdominal part of the body. This maneuver can produce such effects as normalizing the function of the stomach-*qi*, promoting digestion, removing stagnated food, and regulating peristalsis of the intestines.

Rotatory Kneading Maneuver. Using the palmar surface, knead in a rotating manner a certain part or acupoint of the patient's body. The pressure should be gentle and soft at a speed of 120–160 circles per minute. This maneuver provides just a mild stimulation, and it can be applied to any part of the body. The main effects of this maneuver include relieving stuffiness of the chest and regulating the flow of *qi*, promoting digestion, removing stagnated food, activating blood flow, subduing swelling, and alleviating pain.

Mobile Finger-pinching Maneuver. Hold between the finger and the thumb a muscle or tendon of the patient's body; pinch or squeeze tightly and release. Repeat this as many times as necessary. Mobile finger-pinching is usually applied to the thigh, calf, shoulders, or back. It can produce such effects as relieving rigidity of the muscles and dredging the channels and collaterals, promoting the flow of *qi* and activating blood circulation.

Rolling Maneuver. Place the back of your hand on a certain part of the patient's body, and roll the hand back and forth under the drive of the wrist joint. To do this properly, keep the wrist joint relaxed and flex the elbow joint slightly forming an angle of about 120 degrees with the arm and shoulders. The pressure applied should be even, and the manipulation must be harmonious and rhythmic at 120–160 rolls a minute. This maneuver can be applied to the shoulders, back, waist, buttocks, or limbs. The rolling maneuver can produce such effects as relieving rigidity of the muscles and joints, activating the flow of blood, alleviating spasms, promoting the circulation of blood, and helping one to recover from exhaustion.

Rubbing Maneuver. Place the palmar surface of the hand on a certain part of the patient's body and rub back and forth along a certain line. It is important that the exertion of pressure be steady and not interrupted. This maneuver is characterized by mild and warm stimulation. Rubbing promotes the flow of *qi* by warming the channels and collaterals, subduing swelling, and alleviating pain. It also strengthens the spleen and stomach, lifts local temperature of the body, and promoting the circulation of blood and lymph. Palmar rubbing is mostly applied to the abdomen, shoulders, back, waist, and lower limbs.

Clapping Maneuver. Shape your palm like a cup, and clap the body surface of the patient. The clapping should be steady and rhythmic. This maneuver can be applied to the shoulders, back, and lower limbs. It can relieve rigidity of muscles and tendons, activate collaterals, promote the flow of *qi* and blood, alleviate spasms, and help one to recover from exhaustion.

Fingertip-Pressing Maneuver. Press certain areas of the patient's body with one or two fingertips. This maneuver can provide very strong stimulation. This maneuver is usually applied to those areas where there are few and/or thin muscles. It relieves the syndromes of stroke, eases constipation, activates the flow of blood, alleviates pain, and regulates the function of *zang* and *fu* organs.

Pulse-Pressing Maneuver. Press a certain part of the patient's body like a pulsebeat with the fingers or palm. Finger-pressing can be performed with the middle finger or other fingers and is applicable to the face or other parts of the head. Palm-pressing can be performed with one or two palms and is applicable to any part of the body trunk. This maneuver can relax the muscles, activate the circulation of blood, and relieve pain.

3.3.2 SELF-MASSAGE FOR HEALTHCARE

Self-massage is one of the commonly used methods for the preservation of health. It includes local self-massage and general self-massage. Local self-massage refers to massaging a small area, while general self-massage refers to massaging larger areas.

Indication of Self-massage. Local self-massage is usually prescribed to treat local disorders such as pain, numbness, atrophy, and hypofunction of muscles due to invasion of the evils of wind-cold. It can also be applied to treat indigestion and local neuralgia.

General self-massage is mainly employed to prevent diseases or to preserve health, to build up constitutions, and to obtain longevity. It can also be applied to treat diseases.

Methods of Practicing Self-massage. The following is a brief description of general self-massage. This method is particularly applicable for the aged and less able-bodied. The performance includes the following 20 actions.

1. Tapping of the Teeth. Shut the mouth softly and tap the teeth rhythmically 30–40 times.

2. Cleaning of the Mouth. Shut the mouth softly, and wash the surface of the teeth and the teeth ridges with the tongue—from right to left and vice versa, 30 times.

3. Rubbing of the Palms. Rub the palms together energetically until they are warm.

4. Wiping the Face. Wipe the face with the warmed palms from the forehead to the chin, 20–30 times.

5. Combing the Hair. Comb the hair with the ten fingertips of the hands from the forehead backward to the occipital area, 20–30 times.

6. Kneading the Temples. Knead the temples with the tips of the middle fingers in a circular manner clockwise and counterclockwise, 7–8 times.

7. Kneading the Eyes. Knead the eyes around the orbits with the knuckles of the forefingers, middle fingers, and ring fingers—counterclockwise and then clockwise for 7–8 times.

8. Pressing the *Jingming* (UI 1) Points. Press the *Jingming* points with the forefinger tips and then release the tips for a pause. Do this 15–30 times.

9. Pressing the Temples Rotatorily. Press the temples in a clockwise and counterclockwise manner 10–15 times each way.

10. *Ming Tiangu* (Auricular Drilling). Press the ears tightly with the palms while tapping the occiput 15 times with the forefingers, middle fingers, and ring fingers.

11. Kneading the Breasts. Put the palms on the breasts, above the nipples and to the outer sides. Knead in a circular manner in both clockwise and counterclockwise direction, 10 times each.

12. Pinching the Shoulder Muscles. Hold the left shoulder muscle at about the point *Jianjing* with the thumb and the forefinger and the middle finger of the right hand and pinch. Change sides and do the same to the right shoulder muscle with the left hand. Do the above alternately, 10–15 times on each side.

13. Broadening the Chest. Place the hands on either side of the sternum with the fingers slightly apart from each other and move the tips of the fingers along the intercostal spaces from the breastbone to the sides. Do this 10–15 times.

14. Kneading the Abdomen. Knead the abdomen with one hand from the stomach part down the left side of the navel to the lower abdomen, and then return to the starting point by continuing up the right side. Do this 10–15 times.

15. Rubbing the Lumbar Region. Rub the palms together to warm

them and press the lumbar region tightly. Rub this area in an up-and-down manner 30 times.

16. Pressing the *Huantiao* (GE 30) Points. Lie down on the right side with the right leg stretching straight and the left leg flexing. Press the left Huantiao point with the left thumb tip. Change sides and press the corresponding right point with the right thumb tip. Do these alternately, 10 times on each side.

17. Rubbing the Thigh. Hold a thigh tightly between the hands and rub it energetically from the hip to the knee and vice versa for 20 times. Be sure that the strength is evenly exerted. Be sure to do both thighs evenly.

18. Kneading the Calf. Hold a calf tightly between the palms, and knead it energetically in a rotatory fashion. Change to the other calf and do the same as above.

19. Rubbing the *Yongquan* (KL 1) Points. Rub the palms together to warm them up, and then rub the left *Yongquan* point quickly and energetically with the palms until the sole is warmed up. Do the same as above to the other *Yongquan* point.

Breathing. Stand straight with feet shoulder-width apart. Breathe in while raising the head, stretching the waist, and lifting the hands from the belly to the throat. Breathe out uttering *Ha, Ho, Xi, Xu* while lowering the head, stooping down, and letting the hands down from the throat back to the abdomen. Do this three times.

Practice the above exercises in the order they are presented here. Those who are less able-bodied can choose some of the exercises at first and gradually cover them all.

Precautions in Practicing Self-massage.
- Never do self-massage after overeating or when you are hungry.
- Be sure that the place for performing self-massage is ventilated with fresh air.
- As a rule, do self-massage twice a day; once in the morning and again in the evening, for about 20 minutes.
- The amount of massage will varies with individuals.
- Concentrate the mind, calm the feelings, and get relaxed when doing self-massage.
- Eat enough nutritious food, avoid exhaustion, and control your sexual life.
- Keep the skin clean. Be sure to wash your hands before self-massage.
- Nails must be cut short and rounded. Talcum powder can be

used on the skin of the limbs or other parts with much hair to prevent injure to the skin.

• Skin contact is significant. Massage that is done through clothing will not be as effective.

3.3.3 INDICATIONS AND CONTRAINDICATIONS

Indications. Massotherapy can be utilized in internal medicine, surgery, pediatrics, and health protection. It can also be used as an auxiliary treatment when dealing with internal diseases, especially chronic or functional diseases. Self-massage is quite effective in treatment of certain diseases during their acute stage such as protrusion of intervertebral disc, acute sprains, acute mastitis, infantile fever, and indigestion or diarrhea of children. This therapy provides a good method for the prevention of diseases and the preservation of good health and longevity.

Contraindications. Massotherapy should not be performed on infectious diseases, local lesion of malignant tumors, burns, scalds, all contagious and suppurative diseases, tubercular arthritis, serious heart disease, hepatic diseases, serious psychoses, gastric or duodenal perforation, hemorrhagic or other fatal diseases. Additionally, females during menstrual period or pregnancy are cautioned not to massage the abdomen or the lumbosacaral area.

Glossary of Terms

Abdominal Breathing. Also called abdominal respiration. During respiration the abdomen expands naturally during inspiration and contracts during exhalation

Auricles. That portion of the external ear not contained within the head.

Cerebral ischemia. Temporary deficiency of blood supply due to obstruction of circulation in the cerebral region.

Cerebral Anoxia. Without oxygen in the cerebral region.

Cervical Spondylopathy. Any disorder of the vertebrae.

Collaterals. Pathways in which qi and blood are circulated in the human body. Collaterals run transversely and superficially from the meridians.

Dantian. Locations in the body that are able to store and generate qi. The Upper, Middle, and Lower Dantian are located, respectively, between the eyebrows, at the solar plexus, and a few inches below the navel.

Daoyin. Also called Daoyin Massage. A comprehensive exercise that combines specific body posture, breath regulation, and mind concentration with self massage to develop both the physical and energetic aspects of the body.

Dysmenorrhea. Pain associated with menstruation.

Dysphoria. An exaggerated feeling of depression and unrest without apparent cause.

Dyspnea. Difficulty in breathing sometimes accompanied by pain.

Enteritis. Inflammation of the intestines.

Epigastralgia. Pain in the pit of the stomach.

Essence. The most refined part of anything.

Exopathy. Pertaining to a disease originating outside the body.

Expectoration. The process of spitting out saliva or coughing up materials from the air passageways leading to the lungs.

Gastritis. Inflammation of the stomach.

Hypertension A condition in which the patient has a blood pressure higher than that judged to be normal.

Hypochondrium. Part of the abdomen beneath the lower ribs on each side of the epigastrium.

Lower Jiao. Lower portion of the body cavity.

Meridians. Pathways in which qi and blood are circulated in the human body. The meridians, which constitute the main trunks, run longitudinally and within the interior of the body.

Mun-Xi. Breathing technique known as full breathing.

Myopia. Defect in vision also known as nearsightedness.

Qi. The general definition of qi is: universal energy, including heat, light, and electromagnetic energy. A narrower definition refers to the energy circulating in animal or human bodies. A current popular model is that the qi circulating in the human body is bioelectric in nature.

Qigong. Study, research, and /or practices related to qi.

Spermatorrhea. Abnormally frequent, involuntary loss of sperm without orgasm.

Syncope. A transient loss of consciousness due to inadequate blood flow to the brain.

Tinnitus. A subjective ringing in the ears.

Xiphoid Process. The lowest portion of the sternum.

Index

BOOKS FROM YMAA

DVDS FROM YMAA

more products available from . . .

YMAA Publication Center, Inc. 楊氏東方文化出版中心

1-800-669-8892 • info@ymaa.com • www.ymaa.com

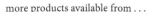

YMAA
PUBLICATION CENTER

Printed in the USA
CPSIA information can be obtained
at www.ICGtesting.com
JSHW022325140824
68134JS00019B/1308

9 781886 969896